D1719992

PAEDIATRIC MASSAGE

Jin Wenlong   Lin Huifang   Wang Shucui
Translated by   He Fei

Morning Glory Publishers   Beijing

Editors: Jiang Cheng'an
    Xu Heng

Translated by He Fei

First edition 1999
ISBN 7-5054-0590-x/G·0168
03000
17-E-3267P

Published by MORNING GLORY PUBLISHERS
   35 Chegongzhuang Xilu, Beijing 100044, China

Distributed by CHINA INTERNATIONAL BOOK
   TRADING CORPORATION
   P.O.Box 399, Beijing
   35 Chegongzhuang Xilu, Beijing 100044, China

Printed in the People's Republic of China

FOREWORD

Massage as medical treatment originated in very early times. It was used in clinics in China more than 2,000 years ago. Easy to practise, convenient, cheap and effective are its features. It is highly welcomed by the masses and particularly by children since massage does not require children to receive injection or take medicine. What's more, massage has no side effects of any kind. A child before going to sleep is in a quiet and relaxed state. The parents have ample time to massage the child without difficulty. We have compiled this book: Paediatric Massage for the benefit of parents (and whoever is interested in massage) so that they may practise massage on the children.

We have chosen 35 common or frequently occurring paediatric diseases suitable for massage treatment. The cause, pathology and symptom are given so that parents can have a general idea of these diseases. We show one or several massage methods that can be applied as treatment in accordance with the condition of the patient. Our clinical experiences tell us that massage for children can not be successful if one merely masters commonly used manipulations or a few ready made prescriptions. Care must be taken to examine the manifestations of diseases while symptoms and signs must be analysed before massage methods are used. To meet this need the book provides detailed exposition on diagnosis of diseases.

In order that parents may pay enough attention to nurse children in an overall manner, we provide nursing care as suggested regimen. In certain emergency cases massage can only be used as a supplementary measure. It is hoped that parents will read carefully the related passages. Necessary information on nursing care is provided. Careful nursing care will prevent or cut down complications, alleviate disease and promote early recovery.

In compiling this book we try to be as simple, explicit and practical as possible so that readers may be able to manipulate massage after reading the text.

The authors

CONTENTS

GENERAL KNOWLEDGE OF PAEDIATRIC MASSAGE

Paediatric massage constitutes an important part of traditional Chinese medical science to prevent and cure paediatric diseases and keep children fit. From birth the child is in a state of growth and development. Its anatomical physiological characteristics are quite different from those of adults. Its pathology and immunization greatly differ from those of adults. To master the science of paediatric massage an overall and comprehensive knowledge of basic knowhow of the features of child organism and child massage manipulation are requisites. Having mastered these we can correctly massage the children to cure sickness.

Characteristics of Child Physiology and Pathology

As a child grows and develops constantly since birth, its anatomy, physiology, pathology and immunization differ from those of the adult. Changes occur in the shape and location of organism as the child gets older. The physiological functions have yet to reach maturity. Chinese physicians through the ages describe this phenomenon as tender visceral organs with inadequate qi or vital energy. Another feature of the physiology of the child is that it is full of vigour and develops very rapidly. The child is therefore always in a state of developing towards maturity in physique, intellectual power and the functions of the viscera. The younger a child is the more quickly it grows. This is reflected in the urgent need of shui gu and jin qi (nutritious materials). The child is said to have a pure yang constitution. Its physiology is summed up as having immature yin or negative element and an immature yang or positive element by ancient Chinese physicians.

The pathological characteristic of paediatric diseases is that a child easily gets sick and sickness progresses quickly. The viscera and qi or vital energy function clearly. The child can easily recover from its illness. But since its viscera are weak and can also dysfunction, the resistance to disease is weak. As the child by itself can not put on more cloth when it is cold or take off its cloth when it is hot, nor can the child exercise self control on its diet when the stomach is full, plus improper nursing, the child will easily fall prey to the six external factors (wind, cold, summer heat, humidity, dryness and fire). Overeating may hurt the child internally. Consequently we see children frequently attacked by diseases such as cold due to external factors and diseases of the lung and spleen. Clinical experiences tell us that cold, cough and indigestion are common with children. Fever and convulsions easily occur. These diseases break out with great frequency. Once afflicted the state of illness of the child will often change. Deficiency and excess may occur. The disease easily aggravates. From being seriously ill the child will become critically ill. On the other hand full of vigour and vitality, the child is agile and makes quick responses to treatment. The cause of its disease is usually rather simple. It is not affected by seven passions like the adult. The child can quickly get well again, given proper care and timely treatment.

Commonly Used Media in Paediatric Massage

To avoid damaging the tender skin of a child during massage or to enhance therapeutic efficacy by means of medicine, a sort of lubricating oil is applied on the hand or part of the body afflicted with disease, known as massage media. We recommend the following as media to be applied by the massagist in accordance with the condition of the sickness:

1. Ginger juice. Chip ginger into pieces and crush them. Apply the juice on the child in winter and spring. Relieving the exterior syndrome with the pungent flavour and warm property of ginger, this media will induce perspiration, warm the middle-Jiao and strengthen the stomach. It relieves indigestion and cures stomach cold, vomit, bellyache or diarrhoea.

2. Scallion juice. Chip scallion into pieces and crush them. Take out the juice and apply it on the child. It induces sweat, drives away exterior cold and helps the yang element in the constitution of the child. If a child suffers from difficult urination due to cold and qi stagnation the scallion juice is good for it.

3. Chinese ilex ointment, made of winter green oil and

vaseline in the ratio of 1:5. It helps subsidence of swelling, kills pain and dissipates cold. It is an effective media for all cases of swelling, pain and chronic injury or pain caused by cold.

4. Break open the shell of an egg. Let the egg white drip down into a cup by putting it upside down with the aid of two wooden sticks. The white of egg does several jobs: dissipate heat, remove indigestion or food accumulation, and relieve feverish sensation in the palms and soles, worry, and sleeplessness after illness.

5. Use fresh or dry peppermint leaf and dip it in boiling water and let it steam inside by placing a lid on the cup for 8 hours. Apply the juice as a media on parts of the body in summer to cure cold or headache due to pathogenic wind-heat, red eyes, sore throat or small pox in the early stage.

6. Talcum powder should be applied to infants or those with tender skin in all seasons of the year.

7. Ordinary spirits in the market can be applied to the body to increase or facilitate the flow of blood and channels, kill pain, end numbness or stasis of blood.

8. Other methods used are: cold water to remove fever; Fengyoujin Essence to cure cold due to wind heat; camphor wine to end muscle pain; and cinnamon oil to cure aversion to cold and weak constitution.

Points for Attention in Paediatric Massage

Put the child in a quiet place with suitable room temperature for massage. High room temperature should be avoided.

Otherwise the child will sweat in the hands, which will adversely affect manipulation. If room temperature is too low the child might catch cold.

The massagist should wash hands clean and make them warm. Long finger nails should be clipped off to avoid hurting the skin of the child. A clean and soft towel is placed on the skin in the course of manipulation. Of course, the towel should be washed after each manipulation.

The child should be placed in such a position that it is in line with the condition of illness, the acupuncture point, and manipulation requirements. The child should be made to feel comfortable in that position. As a rule children below 3 years of age should be held by somebody. Children above 3 can either sit on a couch, lie on back, in prone position, or lie on side.

The massagist must concentrate his/her mind and manipulate with the hands in a suitable manner. Do not exert too much strength at the beginning. Massage lightly and steadily from shallow to deep parts of the body. Make the child adapt itself to the operation. The massagist should adopt a friendly attitude so that the child will co-operate with him/her. Avoid causing fear in the child, which will affect the process of manipulation.

Massage is carried out once a day before the child goes to sleep. A child who is seriously ill should be massaged more than once a day. The treatment lasts a week. If the child does not get well after two or three weeks of treatment, it should be sent to hospital without delay.

Massage is forbidden in the following cases: burn, scald, scratch, or laceration; acute infectious diseases, such as cellulitis, bone tuberculosis, myelitis and inflammatory disease with red skin, malignant tumour or cancer, bone fracture and dislocation.

Manipulations Commonly Used in Paediatric Massage

1. Tui (Pushing) Method

There are three ways to do this: straight pushing, pushing by two fingers in two directions and spiral pushing. Spiral pushing or pushing in circles is known as bu; straight pushing is qing; and pushing up is xie(pushing in the direction of the bottom of the finger). Sometimes bending the fingers and pushing straight is called bu; pushing straight with stretched fingers is xie; pushing up is qing; and pushing down is bu.

a. Straight pushing. Use thumb end lateral fringe, thumb breadth, breadth of index and middle fingers or bottom of fingers to push forward in a straight line on acupoint or other locations. See Diagram 1.

b. Pushing with two thumbs in two directions. Use thumb breadth to push sideways in two directions from acupoint. See Diagram 2.

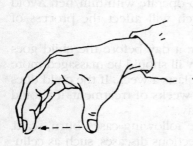

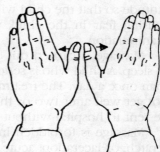

Diagram 1　Straight pushing

Diagram 2　Pushing with two thumbs in two directions

c. Spiral pushing means to push the acupoint with the thumb round and round. See Diagram 3.

2. Yun (Transmitting) Method

Use breadth of thumbs or index, middle and ring fingers to push in arc or circle. It is known as xie if the direction is straight; pu if in opposite direction; han if pushing is done to the left and liang if it is done to the right. Making a left turn is called zhi tu and making a right turn is called zhi xie. See Diagram 4.

3. Rou (Kneading) Method

a. Kneading is done repeatedly in circles with thumb, index finger tip or index, middle and ring finger tips, exerting force on acupoint. See Diagram 5.

b. Kneading with palm. Use the Da and Xiao Yuji (thenar) to knead in circles. See Diagram 6.

c. Kneading with Yuji. This refers to the Da Yuji only,

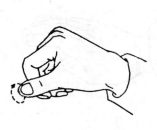

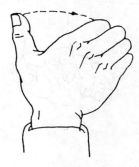

Diagram 3   Spiral pushing   Diagram 4   Thumb Yun method

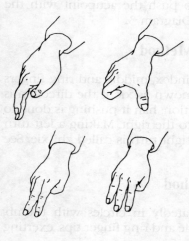

Diagram 5   Kneading with
fingers

which exerts force. It kneads in circles on acupoint. See Diagram 7.

4. An (Pressing) Method

The massagist puts his/her thumb breadth or bottom of palm firmly on the acupoint or desired location and gradually pushes downward with force. Pressing is usually combined with kneading. It is called an rou in Chinese (pressing and kneading).

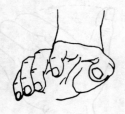

Diagram 6   Kneading with palm

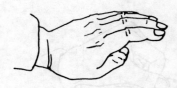

Diagram 7   Kneading with Yuji

8

5. Mo (Rubbing) Method

Mo is a commonly used method in massage for children. It falls into three categories: finger rubbing, palm rubbing and spiral rubbing. Rubbing in the same direction is called Bu. Rubbing in the reverse direction is Xie. Rubbing with palm is Bu. Rubbing with fingers is also Xie. Rubbing in a relaxed manner is also called Bu. Rubbing rapidly is again called Xie.

a. Finger rubbing. Put index, middle and ring fingers on the acupoint or specific location and rub in spiral fashion repeatedly. See Diagram 8.

b. Palm rubbing. Use the palm to do spiral rubbing on the acupoint or desired location. See Diagram 9

c. Spiral rubbing. Exert force with the whole palm and finger breadth of both hands to do spiral rubbing. Begin from the lower belly of the child along the rising part of the colon, transverse colon and the posterior colon. The hands alternate in spiral rubbing: one hand goes in front and the other at the back. See Diagram 10.

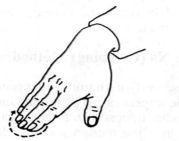

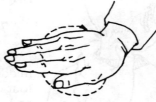

Diagram 8   Finger rubbing   Diagram 9   Palm rubbing

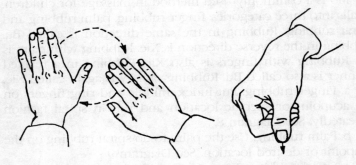

Diagram 10   Spiral rubbing

Diagram 11   Pinching
acupoint with fingernails

6. Qia (Pinching) Method

Let the finger nail of the thumb pinch the acupoint with
force. But do not injure or scratch
the skin. This is a commonly used
method in paediatric massage. See
Diagram 11.

7. Na (Gripping) Method

Use end of thumb, index and
middle fingers or tip of thumb and
four other fingers with force to grip
and pinch the tendon and muscle.
The latter method is also known as
Five-finger Na (Gripping) Method.

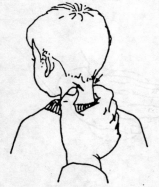

Diagram 12   Na (Gripping) See Diagram 12

8. Nie (Holding Between Fingers) Method

There are two methods under this heading. Holding the skin between fingers and lifting it up is one way. The other way is to hold the skin between thumbs, index, middle and ring finger tips and squeeze it into the centre position by means of kneading from the acupoint or specific location.

   a. In the former case the thumbs and index fingers of both hands should be in a position as if the massagist is grabbing something. The massagist grabs and kneads forward three times the skin from the lumbosacral region along the spinal column to the vertebra (the hands alternate as you go along), lifting up the skin to Dazhui acupoint once. Comb and wipe the skin with the tip of index, middle and ring fingers along spinal column sideways. Each time you grab and knead, you comb and wipe once. During manipulation be careful not to lift up the skin too much or with too much strength. Manipulate in straight line, not slantwise. See Diagrams 13, 14 and 15.

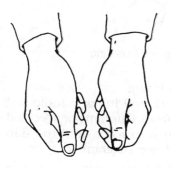

Diagram 13   Manipulating with thumbs and index finger (front view)

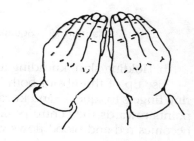

Diagram 14   Holding skin with thumbs and index fingers, etc. (front view)

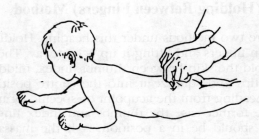

Diagram 15   Gripping spinal column

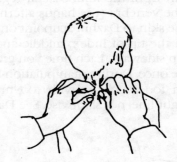

Diagram 16   Squeezing and kneading

b. Holding skin, kneading and lifting

Use tip of thumbs of both hands and index, middle and ring fingers to squeeze and knead from acupoints or specified points towards the centre position with force until the skin becomes red and blood flows well. See Diagram 16.

9. Cuo (Twisting Between Palms) Method

Use the palm of both hands to grip specified parts of the

body with some strength and rub the parts quickly, alternating the hands. Rubbing can also be done simultaneously. Move the hands up and down repeatedly. This is known as Cuo method. See Diagram 17.

10. Ca (Rubbing) Method

Use the outer edge of the thumb or breadth of index, middle and ring fingers to rub forward and backward on acupoint or specific location on the body surface. See Diagram 18. There are three Ca methods—rubbing with fingers, palms and the Yuji acupoints.

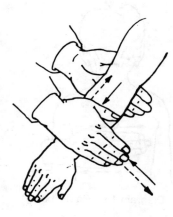

Diagram 17   Twisting between palms

11. Mo (Daubing) Method

Press closely against skin with the breadth of the thumb of one or two hands and move the hands up and down and left and right repeatedly. See Diagram 19.

12. Nian (Twisting) Method

Grip the acupoint or specific position with the breadth of the thumb and index finger and twist and move the acupoint or specific position in a parallel manner with considerable strength. See Diagram 20.

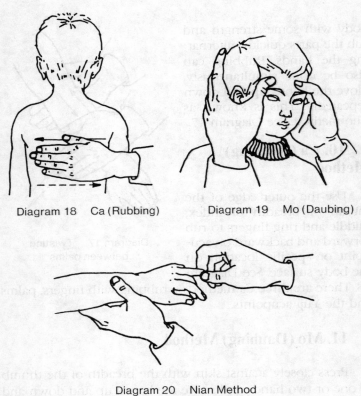

Diagram 18   Ca (Rubbing)

Diagram 19   Mo (Daubing)

Diagram 20   Nian Method

Commonly Used Paediatric Massage Acupoints

In using paediatric massage to cure diseases of children, the massagist should master the commonly used massage methods and acquaint himself/herself with the actual positions of acupoints on the body as well.

1. Methods of Choosing Commonly Used Acupoints

In the course of massage it is important for the massagist to select the right acupoint. The acupoints in the jingmai —main and collateral channels or network of passages are fixed, and so are the qiyue or extra points. There are four ways to ascertain the position.

a. By bone-length measurement. The joints in the body are used as chief landmarks to measure the size and length of various parts of the body in terms of feng cun according to ratio to determine the standard to locate the position of acupuncture. For instance, the traverse crease from wrist to elbow is said to be 12 feng cun. This means that it is divided into 12 sections, which are used as unit of measurement. The commonly used measurement of feng cun is shown in Table 1.

Table 1   Commonly used bone-length feng cun

Position in the body	Starting point to ending point	Commonly used bone-length	Measurement Method
Head	from front hairline to back hairline	12	straight
	between eyebrows to front hairline	3	straight
	back hairline to vertebra	3	straight
	between two processus mastoideus (Wangu acupoint)	9	horizontal
	two sideburns on forehead (Touwei acupoint)	9	horizontal

Chest and belly	Between two nipples	8	horizontal
	belly bottom axilla line to Jilei or 11th rib	12	straight
	From qigu or rib-diaphragm corner to navel	8	straight
	From navel to upper tuberculum pubicum	5	straight
Back	Between inner edge of two shoulder blades	6	straight
	In between posterior superior spine	3	horizontal
Upper	Traverse crease from wrist to elbow	12	straight
Limbs	Traverse crease from elbow to axillar	9	straight
Lower	From big bend of thigh bone to below kneecap	19	straight
Limbs	Below kneecap to high point of outer condylus	16	straight
	Pectineal line to inner condylus of thigh bone	18	straight
	Below inner side of condylus of shin bone to high point of inner condylus	13	straight

b. Locating acupoint by bodily mark

There are two ways to locate acupoint under this method: by fixed marks of the human body or marks formed due to activities of the human body. The former refers to protruding parts or depressions of the five organs—ear, eye, lip, nose and tongue—hair, finger or toe nails, nipple and bone joint or protruding parts of muscle. Activity marks refer to cavity or hole, depression or wrinkle that appear due to movement of joints, muscles and skin, chosen as acupoints.

c. Using a person's finger to locate acupoint means to divide the body into parts.

As the finger of a person is in proportion to other parts of the body, the fingers of the patient are used to measure the body and locate the acupoint. When the middle finger is bent, the two edges of the second segment of the finger are taken as one unit of measurement, called cun. It is described as middle finger versus body cun, which is applied as a horizontal cun to measure limbs and spine or back (Diagram 21). The horizontal length of the thumb joint is taken as one cun, called thumb versus body cun (Diagram 22) to measure four limbs in straight cun measurement to locate the acupoint. Close index, middle, ring and small fingers together. With the second segment of the middle finger as standard, the horizontal length of the four fingers is three cun. This is known as horizontal finger versus body measurement (Diagram 23). It is applied as the horizontal cun to measure lower limbs, lower part of the belly and back of the human body.

d. Easy method of locating acupoint.

Let the tiger mouth or part of the hand between the

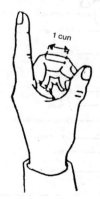

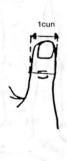

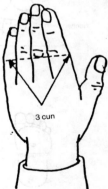

Diagram 21   Middle
finger versus body cun

Diagram 22
Thumb versus
body cun

Diagram 23
Horizontal finger
versus body cun

17

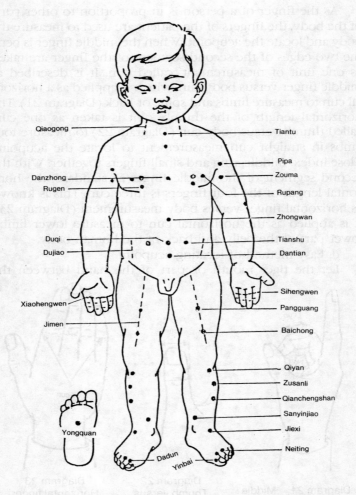

Diagram 24　Distribution of acupoints on whole body (front view)

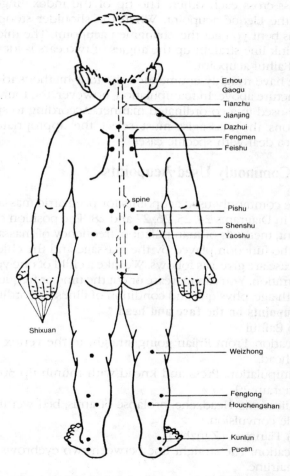

- Erhou
- Gaogu
- Tianzhu
- Jianjing
- Dazhui
- Fengmen
- Feishu

spine

- Pishu
- Shenshu
- Yaoshu

Shixuan

- Weizhong

- Fenglong
- Houchengshan

- Kunlun
- Pucan

Diagram 25　Distribution of acupoints at back of body (hind view)

thumb and index finger hold straight in a natural manner and criss-cross each other. The tip of the index finger becomes the Lieque acupoint. When the shoulder stoops and elbow is bent you get the Zhangmen acupoint. The midpoint in the link line straight up the angles of two ears is identified as the Baihui acupoint.

We have roughly enumerated the four methods to locate acupuncture above. In manipulation, however, the four methods are used in a co-ordinated manner. According to specific conditions the massagist must select the appropriate acupoints to deal with specific cases.

2. Commonly Used Acupoints

The commonly used acupoints for paediatric massage are shown in Diagrams 24, 25, 26, 27 and 28. The position of each acupoint, methods of manipulation, frequency of massage (or time), the function played by the massage and the chief cure for disease are given as follows. We take a child of one year old as illustration. You can increase or cut the time or frequency in line with age, physique and condition of illness accordingly.

Acupoints on the face and head
(1) Baihui
Location: From Erjian going straight to the vertex or top of the head.
Manipulation: Press and knead with thumb tip 30 times. See Diagram 29.
Indications: Headache, prolapse of anus, bed wetting and infantile convulsion.
(2) Tianmen (Zanzhu)
Location: The straight line between two eyebrows to the front hairline.
Manipulation: Push with thumb breadth from eye brows

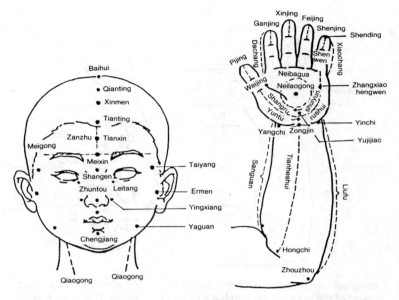

Diagram 26   Acupoints on head, face and neck

Diagram 27   Acupoints on the medial side of the upper limbs and on the palmar aspect

to front hairline 30-50 times. Alternate the thumbs as you operate. See Diagram 30.

Indications: Cold with fever, headache, mental depression and convulsion.

(3) Kangong (Meigong)

Location: The straight line from one end of the brow to tip of brow on the ridge over the eye.

Manipulation: Two thumbs push from the end of the brow to the tip of the brow—one to the left and the other to the right 30-50 times each. See Diagram 31.

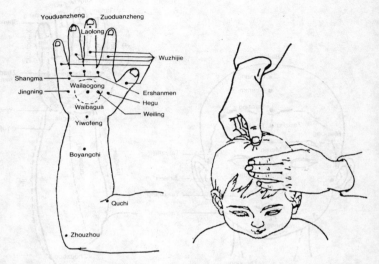

Diagram 28   Acupoints on the posterior aspect of the upper limbs and back of hand

Diagram 29   Press and knead Baihui acupoint

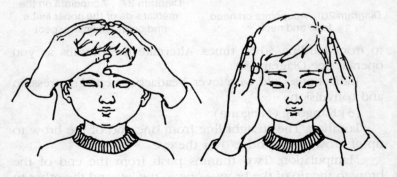

Diagram 30   Pushing Tianmen

Diagram 31   Pushing Kangong

Indications: Cold caused by external factors with fever, headache, red eyes and convulsion.

(4) Taiyang

Location: In the depression behind two eyebrow tips. The Chinese terms are Taiyang for the left side and Taiyin for the right side.

Manipulation: Knead the two acupoints on left and right (Taiyang and Taiyin) with two thumbs or two middle finger tips. Kneading to the front is known as Bu. Kneading to the back of the ear is called Xie. Knead thirty times each. See Diagram 32.

Indications: Cold with fever, headache and dizziness.

(5) Renzhong

Location: On the face at the intersection between the upper third and middle third of the philtrum.

Manipulation: Pinch the acupoint with the nail of the thumb 3 or 5 times. See Diagram 33.

Indications: Coma, infantile convulsion or spasm.

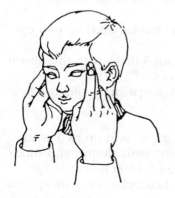

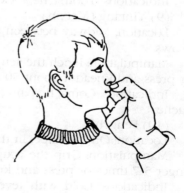

Diagram 32　Kneading Taiyang

Diagram 33　Pinching Renzhong

23

(6) Shangen (Shanfeng)

Location: Between the inner corner of the eye and the depression of the nose bridge (nasal bone).

Manipulation: This acupoint is not for pushing. Pinch it only with your thumb nail 3-5 times.

Indications: Convulsions and spasm.

(7) Yingxiang

Location: About five cun from the wing of nose or ala nasa.

Manipulation: Press and knead the acupoint with index and middle fingers 15-30 times.

Indications: Nasal obstruction, nasal mucus and facial paralysis with wry mouth and slanting eyes.

(8) Yaguan (Jiache)

Location: One cun anterior and superior to the mandibular angle, in the depression where the masseter muscle is prominent.

Manipulation: Press and knead the acupoint with thumbs or middle fingers 15-30 times.

Indications: Toothache, lock jaw and facial paralysis.

(9) Yintang (Meixin)

Location: Midway between the medial ends of two eyebrows.

Manipulation: Pinch the acupoint 5 times with thumbnail or press and knead it about 50 times.

Indications: Coma, tic pain (hyperspasma), cold and headache.

(10) Fengchi

Location: On the nape, in the depression on two sides.

Manipulation: Grip the acupoint with thumb and index finger 5-7 times or press and knead 50-100 times.

Indications: Cold with fever, headache, eyes dizzy and nasal obstruction.

(11) Tianzhu (Tianzhugu)

Location: The straight line between the centre of the nape and the Dazhui acupoint.

Manipulation: Push straight from top to bottom with thumb or index and middle fingers 100-500 times. See Diagram 34.

Indications: Vomit, stiff neck, fever, and infantile convulsions.

(12) Dazhui

Location: Between the 7th cervical vertebra and the spinous process of the 1st thoracic vertebra.

Manipulation: This acupoint should be pressed and kneaded with middle finger tip 100-300 times or pinched and squeezed with thumb, index, middle and ring fingers (using force in an even manner) 10-15 times.

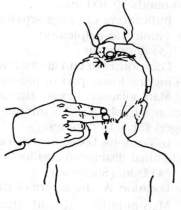

Diagram 34　Pushing Tianzhu with fingers

Indications: Fever, asthma, shoulder and back pain, stiff neck and whooping cough.

Acupoints on the chest and abdomen

(1) Tiantu

Location: In the centre of the supresternal fossa.

Manipulation: Press and knead with thumb or middle finger 15-30 times.

Indications: Asthma, cough, choking sensation in the chest, nausea and vomit.

(2) Danzhong

Location: At the midpoint of the line linking the two

nipples.

Manipulation: Press and knead the acupoint with middle finger tip 50-100 times. Push to the outside from the acupoint outwardly (left and right) with the breadth of the thumb of two hands 50-100 times.

Indications: Choking sensation in the chest, cough, asthma, vomit and palpitation.

(3) Zhongwan

Location: Four cun above navel at the midpoint in the line linking the lower part of the sternum and the navel.

Manipulation: Knead the acupoint with finger tip or bottom of palm for 2-5 minutes or rub it with palm or four fingers for 5-10 minutes.

Indications: Loose bowels or diarrhoea, vomit, bellyache, abdominal distension and loss of appetite.

(4) Duqi (Shenque)

Location: At the centre of the navel.

Manipulation: Knead the acupoint with middle finger tip or bottom of palm 100-300 times.

Indications: Abdominal distension, belly-ache, constipation, diarrhoea and indigestion.

(5) Fu

Location: Abdomen.

Manipulation: Push with thumbs from the xiphoid process along the edge of the arcus costarum to left and right or push from Zhongwan to the navel on left and right.See Diagram 35. Another way is to

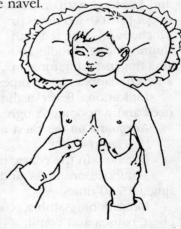

Diagram 35   Pushing the left and right of the abdomen

knead and rub the abdomen clockwise with palm or four fingers to right and left 30-50 times. Rub the abdomen for 2-5 minutes.

Indications: Abdominal distension, belly-ache, vomit and diarrhoea.

(6) Tianshu

Location: Two cun lateral to centre of the navel.

Manipulation: Knead the acupoint with index and middle finger tips. You may apply medicine to the acupoint and knead the acupoint with the medicine.

Indications: Diarrhoea, constipation, abdominal distension, and dysentery.

(7) Dantian

Location: Two-three cun below the navel.

Manipulation: Knead the acupoint with middle finger tip or bottom part of palm 50-100 times. Rub spiral fashion with four fingers for 2-5 minutes.

Indications: Abdominal pain, bed wetting, prolapse of anus, hernia, and lower abdomen pain.

(8) Dujiao

Location: The muscles and tendon on both sides of the navel.

Manipulation: Grip and knead the muscles on both sides of the navel with thumbs plus index and middle fingers in an even manner 3-5 times. See Diagram 36.

Indications: Abdominal pain and loose bowels.

Acupoints on the back, waist and sacrum

(1) Dingchuan

Location: 0.5 cun below the spinous process of the 7th cervical vertebra.

Manipulation: Press and knead the acupoint with thumb or tip of the middle finger about 50 times.

Indications: Bronchial asthma, bronchitis, pain in the

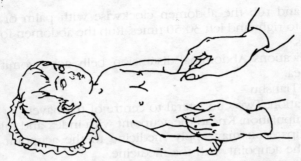

Diagram 36   Gripping and kneading muscles on both
sides of the navel

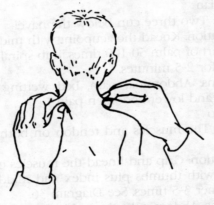

Diagram 37   Pinching and gripping Jianjing

neck and shoulder.

(2) Jianjing

Location: At the midpoint of the line linking Dazhui and acromion, on the muscular part of the shoulder.

Manipulation: Pinch and grip with force muscles on the shoulder about 5-10 times. See Diagram 37.

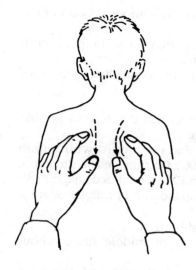

Diagram 38   Pushing Feishu

Indications: Cold, convulsions, pain in the shoulder and pain at the back of the body.

(3) Fengmen

Location: About 1.5 cun below the spinous process of the second thoracic vertebra.

Manipulation: Press and knead the Fengmen acupoints on both sides with the tip of the index and middle fingers about 30 times.

Indications: Cough and asthma.

(4) Feishu

Location: About 1.5 cun below the spinous process of the third thoracic vertebra.

Manipulation: Press and knead the acupoint with index and middle finger tip 15-30 times. Push with two thumbs from the Feishu along the back edge of the shoulder blade downward, 30-50 times each. See Diagram 38.

Indications: Fever, cough and asthma.

(5) Pishu

Location: About 1.5 cun below the spinous process of the 11th thoracic vertebra.

Manipulation: Press and knead the Feishu on both sides with thumbs for 1-3 minutes.

Indications: Diarrhoea, infantile malnutrition, loss of appetite, vomit and weak limbs.

(6) Shenshu

29

Location: About 1.5 cun below the spinous process of the 2nd lumbar vertebra.

Manipulation: Press and knead Shenshu acupoint on both sides with thumbs for 1-3 minutes.

Indications: Bed wetting, frequent micturition, soreness of waist and debility of lumbus.

(7) Qijiegu (Qijie)

Location: The straight line between the second lumbar vertebra and the caudal vertebra.

Manipulation: Push upward and downward with thumb or index and middle fingers 100-500 times each direction. This is known as Shangqijiegu and Xiaqijiegu. See Diagram 39

Indications: Diarrhoea, constipation and prolapse of anus.

(8) Guiwei (Changqiang)

Location: At the tip of the tailbone.

Manipulation: Knead with tip of middle finger about 100-500 times. See Diagram 40.

Indications: Prolapse of anus, constipation and diarrhoea.

(9) Jizhu

Location: Straight line between the Dazhui and tailbone.

Manipulation: Push downward with index and middle finger breadth or bottom of palm about 100-300 times. See

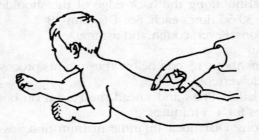

Diagram 39　Pushing Qijiegu

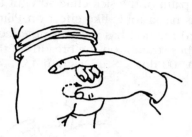

Diagram 40　　Kneading Guiwei

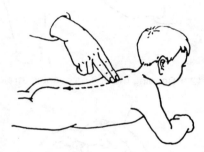

Diagram 41　　Pushing Jizhu

Diagram 41.

Indications: Fever, infantile convulsions, diarrhoea, constipation, infantile malnutrition due to digestive disturbances or intestinal parasites, and other chronic diseases.

Acupoints on the upper limbs

(1) Pijing (Pitu)

Location: Lateral to the radiale of the thumb.

Manipulation: Let the child bend its thumb slightly. The massagist pushes with the breadth of the thumb along the radiale of the palm of the sick child straight to the bottom of the palm. This has a tonic-like effect on Pijing. See Diagram 42. The second method has a cleansing effect on Pijing. The massagist pushes straight on the breadth of the thumb of the sick child 100-300 times. See Diagram 43.

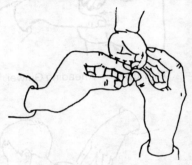

Diagram 42   Bending thumb and pushing straight on Pijing

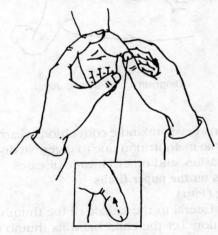

Diagram 43   Cleansing Pijing

Indications: Indigestion, loose bowels, vomit, weak limbs and infantile malnutrition due to digestive disturbances or intestinal parasites.

(2) Ganjing (Ganmu)

Location: On the palmar aspect of the index finger.

Manipulation: Spiral pushing on the palmar aspect of the index finger of the child 100-200 times has a tonic-like effect on the acupoint. Pushing straight from tip to bottom of the index finger 100-300 times will have a cleansing effect. See Diagram 44.

Indications: Infantile convulsions, spasm, red eyes, cold, weak spleen and loose bowels, and hepatitis.

(3) Xinjing (Xinhuo)

Location: On the palmar aspect of the middle finger.

Manipulation: Spiral pushing on the palmar aspect of the middle finger 100-200 times has a tonic-like effect on the acupoint. Pushing straight from the tip to the bottom of the said finger 100-300 times has a cleansing effect. See Diagram 45.

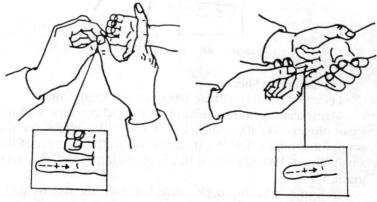

Diagram 44   Pushing Ganjing   Diagram 45   Pushing Xinjing

Indications: High fever, dizziness, fidgeting, crying at night, ulcer in the mouth or tongue, and scanty dark urine.

(4) Feijing (Feijin)

Location: On the palmar aspect of the ring finger.

Manipulation: Spiral pushing on the ring finger 200-400 times has a tonifying effect on the acupoint. Straight pushing from the breadth to the bottom of the ring finger 200-400 times has a cleansing effect. See Diagram 46.

Indications: Fever, cough, asthma, choking sensation in the chest, retropharyngeal abscess and sore throat.

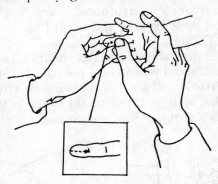

Diagram 46   Pushing Feijing

(5) Shenjing (Shenshui)

Location: On the palmar aspect of the small finger.

Manipulation: Spiral pushing on the palmar aspect of the small finger 200-400 times has a tonic-like effect on the acupoint. Straight pushing from the tip to the bottom of the small finger 100-200 times has a cleansing effect. See Diagram 47.

Indications: Scanty dark urine, bed wetting and frequent micturition.

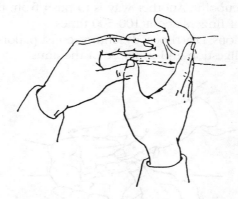

Diagram 47   Pushing Shenjing

(6) Shending
Location: At the tip of the small finger.
Manipulation: Press and knead tip of small finger with thumb 100-300 times.
Indications: Sweating, night sweat and metopism.

(7) Shenwen
Location: In the traverse crease of the first segment on the palmar aspect of the small finger.
Manipulation: Press and knead the traverse crease with the breadth of the thumb about 100-300 times.
Indications: Red eyes, thrush or whitish spots and ulcers on the membranes of the mouth and heat caused by internal factors.

(8) Dachang
Location: Lateral to the radiale of the index finger.
Manipulation: One way is to use index finger tip to push straight to the tiger mouth (part of the hand between the thumb and index finger). This has a tonic-like effect on the

Dachang acupoint. Another way is to push from tiger mouth to the tip of fingers about 100-500 times.

Indications: Diarrhoea, dysentery, constipation, abdominal pain, indigestion and prolapse of the anus.

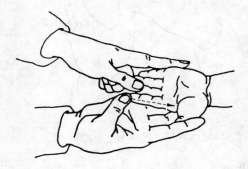

Diagram 48   Pushing Dachang

(9) Xiaochang

Location: Lateral to the radiale of the small finger.

Manipulation: Pushing with thumb straight from the tip to the bottom of the small finger has a tonifying effect on Xiaochang. See Diagram 49. The second way is to push from the bottom to the tip of the small finge to cleanse the acupoint about 100-300 times each way.

Indications: Scanty dark urine, diarrhoea and anure-

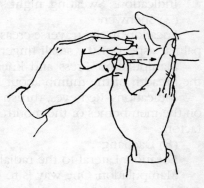

Diagram 49   Pushing Xiaochang

sis.

(10) Sihengwen

Location: In the trav-
erse crease in the joint of
the second segment on
the palmar aspect from
index to small fingers.

Manipulation: Pinch
with the nail of the
thumb the traverse
crease one by one and
knead it about 5-7 times.
See Diagram 50.

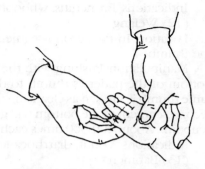

Diagram 50   Pinching Sihengwen

Indications: Abdominal distension, infantile malnutrition,
loss of appetite and asthma.

(11) Xiaohengwen

Location: Lateral to the radiale of the Xiazhangwen at the
bottom of the palmar aspect of the small finger.

Manipulation: Press and knead with the thumb or the tip
of the middle finger on the acupoint about 100-300 times. See
Diagram 51.

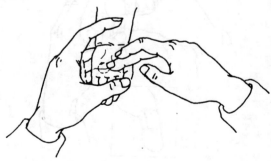

Diagram 51   Kneading Xiaohengwen

Indications: Bronchitis, whooping cough and pneumonia.

(12) Weijing

Location: In the second segment on the palmar aspect of the thumb.

Manipulation: Pushing with the tip of the thumb from the bottom of the patient's thumb to the second segment of the same thumb is known as cleansing the acupoint. Pushing from second segment to the bottom will give a tonifying effect to the acupoint. About 100-300 times each way. See Diagram 52.

Indications: Vomit, diarrhoea and loss of appetite.

(13) Banmen

Location: On the Dayujie of the palm.

Manipulation: Press and knead Dayuji with the tip of the thumb 200-400 times. See Diagram 53.

Indications: Loss of appetite, weak limbs, food retention in the stomach, diarrhoea and abdominal distension.

(14) Xiaotianxin (Yujijiao)

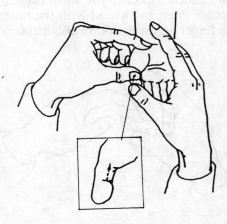

Diagram 52   Pushing Weijing

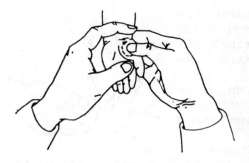

Diagram 53   Kneading Banmen

Location: In the de-
pression between Dayuji
and Xiaoyuji.

Manipulation: Pinch
the acupoint with thumb
nail or knead it with the
tip of the middle finger
30-50 times. See Dia-
gram 54.

Indications: Infantile
convulsions, spasm, fidgeting, dark and difficult urination, red and swollen
eyes with pain.

(15) Neilaogong

Location: In the mid-
dle of the palm to which
the middle and ring fin-
gers point when you bend

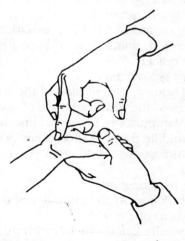

Diagram 54   Pinching and
kneading Xiaotianxin

the fingers.

Manipulation: Press and knead with middle finger tip or the thumb about 50-100 times. See Diagram 55.

Indications: Fever, dry mouth, thirst and other diseases caused by heat.

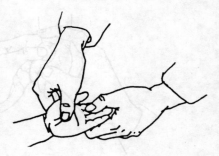

Diagram 55   Kneading Neilaogong

(16) Neibagua

Location: In areas surrounding Neilaogong in the palm of the hand.

Manipulation: Massage with thumb or middle finger clockwise 50-100 times. This operation is called Yun Neibagua. See Diagram 56.

Indications: Choking sensation in the chest, abdominal distension, vomit, loss of appetite and ejecting phlegm not very quickly.

(17) Yiwofeng

Location: On the side of the back of the wrist and in the centre of the traverse crease of the wrist.

Manipulation: Press and knead with thumb or the tip of the middle finger 50-100 times. See Diagram 57.

Indications: Abdominal pain, cold and infantile convulsions.

(18) Zongjing

Location: At the midpoint of the traverse crease lateral to the palm of the wrist.

Manipulation: Pinch it with the tip of the thumb 3-5 times or knead it 10-50 times with the tip of the middle finger.

Indications: Infantile convulsions, spasm, ulcer in the

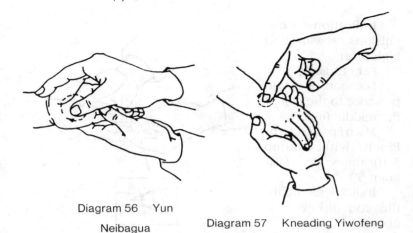

Diagram 56　Yun
Neibagua

Diagram 57　Kneading Yiwofeng

mouth or tongue, toothache and all sorts of diseases caused by excessive heat.

(19) Dahengwen

Location: In the traverse crease at the back of the hand.

Manipulation: Push from Dahengwen with the breadth of the thumb to the left and right 100-300 times. See Diagram 58.

Indications: Abdominal distension, retention of food in the stomach, loose bowels, fidgeting, and asthma.

(20) Shiwang (Shixuan)

Location: At the tip of the ten fingers.

Manipulation: Pinch with thumb nail 5-10 times.

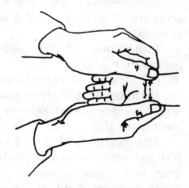

Diagram 58　Pushing left and
right on Dahengwen

Indications: Convulsions, spasm and high fever.

(21) Laolong

Location: 0.1 cun posterior to the nail of the middle finger.

Manipulation: Pinch with thumb 5-10 times. See Diagram 59.

Indications: Infantile convulsions and dizziness.

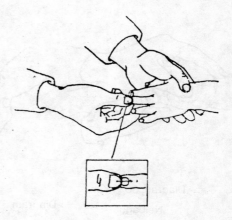

Diagram 59 Pinching Laolong

(22) Ershanmen

Location: In the depression on both sides at the bottom of the middle finger at the back of the hand.

Manipulation: With the nails of two thumbs pinch the acupoint 5-10 times and knead it 100-300 time. See Diagram 60.

Indications: Infantile paralysis, coma and fever without perspiration.

(23) Hukou or Tiger Mouth (Hegu)

Location: In the depression between thumb and index finger on the radial side of the midpoint of the second metacarpal bone.

Manipulation: Press and knead the acupoint with thumb 100-300 times or grip it with thumb and index finger 3-5 times in a parallel manner.

Indications: Cold or disease caused by wind-cold, wry mouth and slanting eyes as well as toothache.

(24) Erma (Shangma, Liangrenshangma)

Location: Between 4th and 5th metacarpal bones at the back of the hand and in the depression behind the finger joint.

Manipulation: Knead the acupoint with thumb or middle finger tip 100-300 times. Pinch it with the nail of the thumb 3-5 times. See Diagram 61.

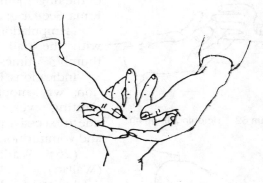

Diagram 60   Pinching Ershanmen

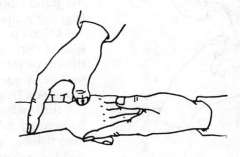

Diagram 61   Kneading Erma

Indications: Scanty and dark urine, infantile convulsions, spasm, weak in health with asthma, and toothache.

(25) Jingning

Location: Between 4th and 5th metacarpal bones at the back of the hand in the depression of the finger joint above Erma. See Diagram 62.

Manipulation: Pinch with the nail of the thumb 3-5 times.

Indications: Indigestion, wry mouth and slanting eyes, asthma due to excessive phlegm, and vomiturition.

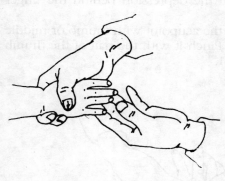

Diagram 62   Pinching Jingning

(26) Wailaogong (Wailao)

Location: In the centre at the back of the hand opposite Neilaogong acupoint.

Manipulation: Knead it with the thumb or the tip of the middle finger 50-100 times. See Diagram 63.

Indications: Cold, bellyache, abdominal distension, diarrhoea and borborygmus.

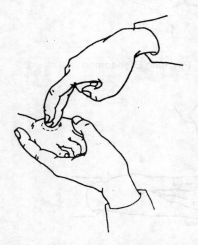

Diagram 63   Kneading Wailaogong

(27) Waibagua

Location: Around Wai-laogong at the back of the hand, opposite Neibagua.

Manipulation: Massage the acupoint clockwise or counter clockwise with the thumb or the middle finger 50-100 times.

Indications: Choking sensation in chest, abdominal distension and constipation.

(28) Sanguan

Location: Lateral to the radiale of the forearm and on the line connectng the traverse crease of the wrist and that of the elbow.

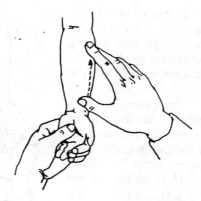

Diagram 64   Pushing Sanguan

Manipulation: Push from the traverse crease of the wrist to that of the elbow with the thumb or the index and middle fingers 100-300 times. See Diagram 64.

Indications: Fever, aversion to cold, anhidrosis, and forearm pain.

(29) Tianheshui

Location: At the centre on the medial side of the forearm and on the line linking the traverse crease of the wrist and that of the elbow.

Manipulation: Push the acupoint from the traverse crease of the wrist to that of the elbow with the index and middle fingers about 100-500 times. See Diagram 65.

Indications: Fever, fidgeting, thirsty, ulcer in mouth and tongue, infantile convulsions and all sorts of diseases due to excess heat.

(30) Liufu

Location: On the ulnar side of the forearm and on the line linking the elbow joint and the traverse crease of the wrist.

Manipulation: Push with the breadth of the thumb or the breadth of the index and middle fingers from the elbow to the wrist about 100-500 times. See Diagram 66.

Indications: All sorts of diseases caused by excess heat, high fever, fidgeting, swelling of throat and pharyngalgia, hard and dry stools, thrush (fungous blisters in the mouth and throat), and mumps.

Acupoints on the lower limbs

(1) Jimen

Location: On the medial side of the thigh and on the line linking the upper part of the kneecap and the groin.

Manipulation: Push straight from inside the

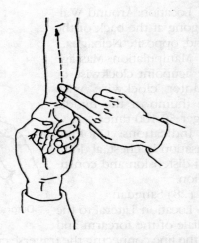

Diagram 65   Pushing Tianheshui

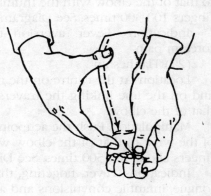

Diagram 66   Pushing Liufu

46

upper part of the kneecap to the groin about 100-300 times. See Diagram 67.

Indications: Scanty dark urine and urinary retention.

(2) Xuehai (Baichong)

Location: With the knee flexed, on the medial side of the thigh, two cun above the superior medial corner of the patella.

Manipulation: Knead it with the tip of the thumb 10-30 times or pinch and lift it up with the thumb, index and middle fingers 3-5 times. See Diagram 68.

Indications: Spasm with twitching of arms and legs, atrophy and weak lower limbs.

(3) Zusanli

Location: Three cun below the knock knee, one finger breadth from the anterior crest of the tibia.

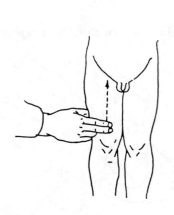

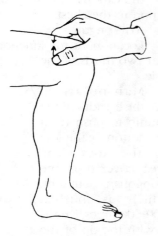

Diagram 68   Holding firmly and
lifting up Baichong

Diagram 67   Pushing Jimen

Manipulation: Press and knead the acupoint with the tip of the thumb for about 1-3 minutes.

Indications: Abdominal distension and pain, loss of appetite, diarrhoea, constipation and weak limbs.

(4) Sanyinjiao

Location: Three cun above the entocondyle.

Manipulation: Press and knead the acupoint with the thumb or the tip of the middle finger for about 1-3 minutes.

Indications: Bed wetting, infantile convulsions and abdominal pain.

(5) Fenglong

Location: Eight cun above the external malleolus, about one finger breadth lateral to Tiaokou.

Manipulation: Knead the acupoint with the thumb or the tip of the middle finger for about 1-3 minutes.

Indications: Excessive phlegm, asthma and choking sensation in the chest.

(6) Yongquan

Location: At the junction of the anterior third and posterior two thirds of the sole.

Manipulation: Use the breadth of the thumb to push from the bottom of the sole to the toes. The area covered is the Yongquan acupoint, which is pushed 100-500 times. Knead it with the tip of the thumb 30-50 times. See Diagram 69.

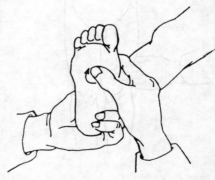

Diagram 69   Kneading Yongquan

Indications: Fever, vomit, diarrhoea and heat sensation in the chest, palms and soles.

3. Other Commonly Used Acupoints

(1) Zhongfu

Location: One cun outside the collarbone.

Indications: Bronchitis, pneumonia, abdominal distension and pain in the chest.

(2) Yunmen

Location: In the depression below the outer extreme point of the collar bone.

Indications: Cough, asthma, irritable and feverish sensation in the chest, and pain in the shoulder and back.

(3) Chize

Location: In the cubital crease and the depreesion of the radial side of the tendon of the biceps muscle of the arm.

Indications: Cough, pharyngalgia, chest stuffiness and hectic fever.

(4) Yuji

Location: At the midpoint of the first metacarpal bone and the junction of the red and white skin.

Indications: Cough, fever, asthma, pharyngalgia and aphonia.

(5) Shaoshang

Location: On the radial side of the thumb, about 0.1 cun from the corner of the finger nail.

Indications: Cough, asthma, fever, coma and pharyngalgia.

(6) Shangyang

Location: On the radial side of the index finger about 0.1 cun from the corner of the finger nail.

Indications: Pharyngalgia, toothache in the lower jaw, coma, cough, and asthma.

(7) Shousanli

Location: With the elbow flexed, two cun below the Quchi acupoint.

Indications: Abdominal distension, aphonia, numbness of hand, and toothache.

(8) Quchi

Location: With the elbow flexed at the lateral end of the cubital crease.

Indications: Pain in the joint of the upper limbs, high fever, eyes becoming red and in pain, and hemiphegic paralysis.

(9) Jianyu

Location: Below acromion on the collar bone, in the depression formed when you raise your forearm level with the shoulder.

Indications: Pain in the shoulder and the arm, hemiparalysis, and nettle rash.

(10) Tianding

Location: At the posterior border at the midpoint of the sterno cleidomastoid muscle.

Indications: Pharyngalgia and aphonia.

(11) Chengqi

Location: When you look straight ahead it is below the pupil and between the eye ball and the infraorbital ridge.

Indications: Myopia, conjunctivitis, night blindness and paralysis of the face.

(12) Sibai

Location: 0.3 cun right below Chengqi in the depression of the infraorbital foramen.

Indications: Red, itchy and painful eyes, shedding tears, and facial paralysis.

(13) Dicang

Location: On the face, directly below the pupil, beside the mouth angle.

Indications: Paralysis of the face, drivelling, toothache and swollen cheek.

(14) Xiaguan

Location: On the face, anterior to the ear, in the depression between the zygomatic arch and the manidibular notch.

Indications: Toothache, tinnitus, deafness and paralysis of the face.

(15) Touwei

Location: 4.5 cun beside the mid hairline at the corner of the forehead.

Indications: Headache, paralysis of facial nerve and dizziness.

(16) Shuidao

Location: Three cun right underneath Tianshu and two cun beside Guanyuan.

Indications: Distension in the lower abdomen, hernia and difficulty in urination.

(17) Futu

Location: Six cun above the upper edge of the kneecap along the line linking the anterior superior iliac spine and lateral edge of the kneecap. You may identify the acupoint when the patient lies on his/her back.

Indications: Paralysis of lower limbs or limbs in partial numbness and pain.

(18) Liangqiu

Location: Two cun above the superiorlateral corner of the kneecap.

Indications: Gastroenteritis (acute and chronic), pain in

knee joint, stomachache and paralysis of lower limbs.

(19) Dubi

Location: In the depression outside the ligamentum patellae below the kneecap (as you bend knee).

Indications: Pain in knee joint and Hong Kong foot.

(20) Shangjuxu

Location: Three cun beneath Zusanli.

Indications: Abdominal pain, borborygmus, dysentery, diarrhoea, constipation, and paralysis resulting from stroke.

(21) Jiexi

Location: At the midpoint of the traverse crease of the ankle joint between the two tendons or sinews, on a par with the tip of the external malleolus.

Indications: Headache, face becoming red, and pain in the ankle joint.

(22) Neiting

Location: On the instep of the foot proximal to the web margin between second and third toes.

Indications: Stomach pain, pharyngalgia, abdominal distension, dysentery, diarrhoea, constipation, swelling and pain in instep of foot.

(23) Yinlingquan

Location: In the depression below the edge of the tibia on the lower border of the medial condyle of the tibia.

Indications: Edema, difficulty in urination, abdominal distension, and pain in kidney and leg.

(24) Shenmen

Location: On the traverse crease of the wrist, in the depression on the radial side of the tendon of the musculus flexor or carpi ulnaris.

Indications: Heart trouble, insomnia, amnesia and pain in wrist joint.

(25) Tinggong

Location: It is a depression between the tragus and the lower jaw joint as you open your mouth.

Indications: Tinnitus, deafness, tympanitis and toothache.

(26) Jingming

Location: 0.1 cun beside the inner canthus.

Indications: Myopia, blurring of image, eyes swollen, red and painful.

(27) Jueyinshu

Location: 1.5 cun below the spinous process of the 4th thoracic vertebra, lateral to the posterior midline.

Indications: Cardiac pain, palpitation, choking sensation in the chest, cough and vomit.

(28) Xinshu

Location: 1.5 cun below the spinous process of the fifth thoracic vertebra lateral to the posterior midline.

Indications: Epilepsy, palpitation with fear, insomnia, cardiopalmus, amnesia, vexation, and cardiac pain.

(29) Geshu

Location: 1.5 cun below the spinous process of the 7th thoracic vertebra lateral to the posterior midline.

Indications: Stomachache, vomit, hiccups, cough and asthma, spitting blood, hectic fever, night sweat, and pain in the back.

(30) Ganshu

Location: 1.5 cun below the spinous process of the 9th thoracic vertebra lateral to posterior midline.

Indications: Hypochondriac pain, red eyes, blurred vision, giddiness, night blindness, mental disorder and pain in spinal column.

(31) Danshu

Location: 1.5 cun below the spinous process of the 10th thoracic vertebra, lateral to the posterior midline.

Indications: Jaundice, bitter taste, pharyngalgia and hypochondriac pain.

(32) Weishu

Location: 1.5 cun below the spinous process of the 12th thoracic vertebra, lateral to the posterior midline.

Indications: Epigastric pain, abdominal distension, vomit, borborygmus, diarrhoea, and indigestion.

(33) Sanjiaoshu

Location: 1.5 cun below the spinous process of the 1st lumbar vertebra, lateral to the posterior midline.

Indications: Abdominal distension, borborygmus, dysentery, difficulty in urination and edema.

(34) Dachangshu

Location: 1.5 cun below the spinous process of the 4th lumbar vertebra, lateral to the posterior midline.

Indications: Abdominal pain and distension, borborygmus, diarrhoea, constipation, and pain in the hip and back.

(35) Guanyuanshu

Location: 1.5 cun below the spinous process of the 5th lumbar vertebra, lateral to the posterior midline.

Indications: Abdominal distension, diarrhoea, bed wetting, urinary obstruction, and diabetes.

(36) Xiaochangshu

Location: On the sacrum and on the level of the 1st posterior sacral foramen, 1.5 cun lateral to the medial sacral crest.

Indications: Bed wetting, hematuria, distension and pain in the lower abdomen, diarrhoea, dysentery and hernia.

(37) Pangguangshu

Location: On the sacrum and on the level of the 2nd posterior foramen, 1.5 cun lateral to the medial sacral crest.

Indications: Difficulty in urination, dark urine, bed wetting, diarrhoea and hip pain.

(38) Baliao

Location: There are eight acupoints on the left and right of the first, second, third and fourth posterior sacral foramina, known as Shangliao, Ciliao, Zhongliao and Xialiao respectively. Taken together they are referred to as Bailiao (eight liao).

Indications: Infection in the urinary tract and prolapse of the anus.

(39) Weizhong

Location: At the midpoint of the popliteal crease.

Indications: Pain in the waist and back, pain in the joint of the knee, systremma, acute gastroenteritis and atrophy of lower limbs.

(40) Chengshan

Location: Beneath gastrocnemius muscle belly—at the skew angle when you stretch your leg.

Indications: Pain in the leg, spasm of gastrocinemius, piles, constipation, hernia, and abdominal pain.

(41) Kunlun

Location: In the depression between the Achilles tendon and the tip of the outer ankle.

Indications: Headache, stiff neck, giddiness and epilepsy.

(42) Shenmai

Location: In the depression right below the outer ankle.

Indications: Epilepsy, headache, dizziness, insomnia, red eyes, ophthalmodynia, and stiff neck.

(43) Taixi

Location: In the depression between inner ankle and the Achilles tendon.

Indications: Headache, dizziness, pharyngalgia, toothache, tinnitus, deafness, insomnia, amnesia, and swelling and pain in inner ankle.

(44) Neiguan

Location: Two cun on the crease of wrist between the tendons of the long palmar muscle palmaris and radial flexor muscle of the wrist.

Indications: Cardiac pain, palpitation, stomachache, vomit, hiccup, insomnia and chest pain.

(45) Waiguan

Location: Two cun proximal to the dorsal crease of the hand.

Indications: Headache, swelling, red eyes and ophthalmodynia, tinnitus, fever, hypochondriac pain and numbness.

(46) Yifeng

Location: Behind the earlobe, in the depression between the corner of lower jaw and mastoid process.

Indications: Tinnitus, deafness, wry mouth and slanting eyes, and swelling cheek.

(47) Ermen

Location: Anterior to the supratragic notch, in the depression behind the posterior border of the condyloid process of the mandible.

Indications: Deafness, tinnitus, otitis media and toothache.

(48) Sizhukong

Location: In the depression of the lateral end of the eyebrow.

Indications: Headache, facial paralysis and eye disease.

(49) Tongziliao

Location: 0.5 cun lateral to the outer canthus.

Indications: Headache, ophthalmodynia and epiphora induced by wind.

(50) Tinghui

Location: Anterior to the intertragic notch in the depression posterior to the condyloid process of the mandible when you open your mouth.

Indications: Tinnitus, deafness, toothache, facial paralysis, and headache.

(51) Yangbai

Location: One cun above the midpoint of the eyebrow.

Indications: Headache, dizziness, ophthalmodynia and night blindness.

(52) Fengchi

Location: Between the upper ends of the sternocleidomastoid trapezius muscles, on a par with Fengfu.

Indications: Cold, headache, fever and pain in shoulder and back.

(53) Huantiao

Location: At the junction of the middle third and lateral third of the line linking the highest point of the great trochanter and the sacral hiatus when you lie on your side with bent legs.

Indications: Hemiparalysis, nettle rash all over the body and pain in waist and hip.

(54) Yanglingquan

Location: In the depression anterior and inferior to the head of the fibula.

Indications: Paralysis of lower limbs, pain in knee joint, numbness, infantile convulsions, pain in the hypochondriac and costal region.

(55) Guangming

Location: About 5 cun right above the tip of outer ankle.

Indications: Ophthalmodynia, night blindness, pain in the knee and flaccid paralysis in the lower limbs.

(56) Qiuxu

Location: In the depression anterior and inferior to outer ankle.

Indications: Flaccid paralysis in the lower limbs, swelling and pain in the outer ankle, hernia, pectoralgia, hypochondriac pain, and apoplectic paralysis.

(57) Juegu

Location: Three cun above tip of the outer ankle.

Indications: hemiparalysis, distension and fullness in the chest and abdomen, gonyalgia and leg pain.

(58) Taichong

Location: In the depression distal to the junction of the first and second metatarsal bones.

Indications: Headache, dizziness, hernia, infantile convulsions, hypochondriac pain, swollen red eyes, ophthalmodynia, and atrophy and paralysis in the lower limbs.

(59) Zhangmen

Location: Beneath the free end of the 11th rib.

Indications: Abdominal distension and pain, borborygmus, diarrhoea, pectoraligia, hypochondriac pain and vomit.

(60) Qimen

Location: In the 6th rib beneath the nipple.

Indications: Pectoralgia, hypochondriac pain, vomit, hiccup, abdominal distension, hungry but with no desire to eat, irritable and feverish sensation in the chest.

(61) Zhongji

Location: Four cun below the navel.

Indications: Bed wetting, infection of the urinary tract and hernia.

(62) Qihai

Location: 1.5 cun below the navel.

Indications: Abdominal pain, diarrhoea, prolapse of anus, bed wetting and weak limbs.

(63) Shuifen

Location: One cun above the navel.

Indications: Edema, difficulty in urination, abdominal pain and borborygmus.

(64) Jianli

Location: Three cun above the navel.

Indications: Abdominal distension and pain, vomit, edema, and loss of appetite.

(65) Lianquan

Location: Above Adam's apple, in the depression of the upper border of the hyoid bone.

Indications: Swelling and pain in the lower part of the tongue, stiff tongue, aphasia resulting from stroke, laryngitis, mouth parched and tongue scorched, deaf and dumb and diabetes.

(66) Chengjiang

Location: At the midpoint of the groove between lower lip and chin.

Indications: Toothache, wry mouth, slanting eye and gum-boil.

(67) Mingmen

Location: In the depression below the spinous process of the second lumbar vertebra.

Indications: Bed wetting, frequent urination, diarrhoea, dizziness, tinnitus, and fright.

(68) Zhiyang

Location: In the depression beneath the spinous process of the 7th thoracic vertebra.

Indications: Chest-hypochondrium pain and swelling, abdominal pain, cough and asthma, stiff spine, and fever.

(69) Yamen

Location: 0.5 cun directly above the midpoint of posterior hairline, at the back of the neck.

Indications: Loss of voice, headache, mental disorder and vomit.

(70) Fengfu

Location: One cun directly above the midpoint of the posterior hairline, at the back of the head.

Indications: Headache and diseases of the neck.

(71). Yuyao

Location: At the midpoint of the eyebrow.

Indications: Short-sightedness, conjunctivitis, facial paralysis and ptosis.

(72) Bitong

Location: At the upper end of the groove between the nose and lip.

Indications: Rhinitis and ulcer in parts of the nose.

PAEDIATRIC MASSAGE

Common Cold

Common cold is a disease that frequently occurs among children. The Chinese term for it is *shangfeng*. It is an illness either caused by wind-cold or wind-heat. The commonly seen symptoms are: aversion to cold, fever, headache, nasal obstruction, running nose, pharyngalgia and cough. In serious cases high fever, fidget (morbid restlessness), drowsiness (somnolence), even spasm or convulsions occur.

Massage Method One

1. Commonly used manipulations

a. The child should be held in the arm by the parent or lie on its belly. Use ginger juice to rub two Pangguangjing acupoints along the spinal column. Exert force to push and rub with Dayuji on the back and the hip until the skin becomes red and warm.

b. Press and knead with the thumb of both hands Fengmen and Feishu on the back (one minute for each acupoint).

c. Let the sick child lie on its back. The parent pushes the two wings of the nose or ala nasi with the thumb of both hands 20-30 times respectively. Push Yintang and Zanzhu.

Rub the forehead posterior to Taiyang on the left and right. Repeat the process several times until the skin is slightly red or pink.

d. Press and knead Quchi and Hegu with thumb for 1-3 minutes each.

2. Additional manipulations

a. Common cold caused by wind-cold. The disease aggravates with aversion to cold, light fever, no perspiration, headache, pain in joints of limbs, nasal obstruction, coughing up few phlegm, tongue becoming pale with thin and white coating. Push heavily Sanguan 500 times. Knead Wailaogong 100 times. Hold firmly and lift up the muscular parts of Jianjing with both hands 5-7 times. Quickly knead Ershanmen 50 times with index and middle fingers, using little force.

b. Common cold caused by wind-heat. Fever is high, slight aversion to wind or cold, pharyngalgia, dry mouth, perspiration, red face, nasal obstruction, yellow nasal discharge, coughing up yellow phlegm and the tip of tongue red and coated tongue thin and yellow. Cleanse Feijing 300 times and Tianheshui 100 times; press and knead Dazhui for 1-3 minutes; rub with palm the sacrococcygeal region horizontally till diathermancy; and hold firmly and lift up Jianjing 3-5 times.

c. Press and knead Tiantu and Fenglong for one minute each in case the patient coughs up a lot of phlegm. Push Xiaohengwen and Danzhong 100 times each.

d. Cleanse Feijing and Xinjing 300 times each, push Yongquan 200 times and cleanse Tianheshui 500 times, when you find the patient is in high fever and convulsions.

e. In case the patient suffers from loss of appetite, knead Banmen 100 times; rub Zhongwan for 3 minutes; and press and knead Zusanli for one minute.

Massage Method Two

1. Commonly used manipulations

a. Let the patient lie on his or her back. The parent uses thumb of both hands to rub from Yintang to the front hairline 30 times in an alternate manner. Rub from the centre of the forehead to Taiyang on either side 30 times. Press and knead Taiyang for 1-3 minutes.

b. Knead Yiwofeng for 1-3 minutes.

c. Knead Yingxiang 15-20 times.

d. The parent rubs horizontally the shoulder and back of the child (who lies on its back in bed) till diathermancy.

e. Grip and knead the muscles of upper and lower limbs 3-5 times with thumb and four fingers in an even manner. Rub each position with palm.

2. Additional manipulations

a. In case there are serious nasal discharge and pharyngalgia, press and knead Quchi and Hegu for one minute each. Knead Taiyang as much as possible.

b. In case of high fever, cleanse Tianheshui and Feijing 300 times each. Push the spinal column 5-10 times in a straight manner. Rub Yongquan 300 times.

c. For patients with weak spleen and stomach plus loss of appetite, massage the Pijing acupoint 100 times for tonifying purpose; push Sanguan 100 times; and press and knead Zhongwan and Zusanli for one minute each.

Suggested Regimen

a. See to it that the sick child should lie in bed and have proper rest in a room that is clean, provided with fresh air and adequate humidity, and dustless. Dry air should be avoided. If the room is too dusty it will affect the nose and throat and make the child cough.

b. Semi-liquid food, lightly seasoned, is recommended for the child during the period of sickness, such as egg soup and millet congee. No greasy food should be taken. Let the child drink a lot of water and eat green vegetables and fruits.

c. Cold or flu during the period of sickness may give rise to complications, such as pneumonia, tympanitis, etc. If complications arise consult the doctor.

Cough

Cough is a commonly seen symptom in child disease. It occurs in all seasons of the year but more often in winter and spring. There are two categories of cold as shown by clinical experience: cough caused by cold due to external factors and cough due to internal injury or disorder of the internal organ. The more commonly seen cough among children is cough caused by external factors, accompanied by fever, nasal obstruction, choking sensation in the chest, shortness of breath, dry cough with little or lots of phlegm as well as mental fatigue.

Massage Method One

1. Commonly used manipulations
a. Let the child lie on its belly. The parent uses Xiaoyuji to press and knead Feishu at the back of the child for five minutes, followed by pushing the shoulder blade on both sides 100 times.

b. Let the child lie on its back. Press and knead Tiantu with thumb 50 times and knead Danzhong for one minute.

c. Press, knead, whisk and pluck Zusanli and Fenglong for one minute each.

2. Additional manipulations

a. When the child suffers from wind-cold due to external factors (with symptoms such as cough, scanty but white phlegm, nasal obstruction, running nose, itching of pharynx, pain in head and body, fever, aversion to cold, no perspiration, and thin and white tongue coating), push Sanguan 300 times, lift up Fengchi and Hegu 10 times each or push Taiyang 10 times as added treatment.

b. In the case of cold due to wind-heat caused by external factors (with symptoms such as cough, yellow phlegm, crackling sound and difficulty in respiratory organs, dry pharynx and pharyngalgia, or chest pain, fever and sweat plus thin yellow coated tongue), cleanse Feijing and push Liufu 300 times each, knead Dazhui 30 times, press and knead Jianjing 10 times, and lift up Jianjing with thumb of both hands as well as index and middle fingers 5 times.

c. For cough described as of wet phlegm, with repeated cough, coughing up lots of white phlegm, choking sensation in chest, nausea and white greasy coated tongue, massage Pijing 300 times for cleansing purpose, pinch and knead Sihengwen 5 times and Yun (transmit) Neibagua 100 times.

d. For cough of fire-heat type with repeated dry cough, scanty phlegm with blood streak, distending pain in chest and hypochondria, fidgeting and bitter taste, red face and eyes, red border of tongue, thin and yellow tongue coating and lack of saliva, press and knead Xiaohengwen 100 times, knead Neilaogong 50 times, push Yongquan 200 times and knead Shenshu for one minute.

Massage Method Two

a. Press and knead Danzhong for 2 minutes.

b. Let the child lie on its back. The parent stands in front of the head of the child. He/she places thumbs on the head with other four fingers being stretched out. Push from breast bone along the first to the fourth ribs outwardly to the mid axillary line for three minutes.

c. Let the child lie on the belly. The parent presses and kneads Feishu and Pishu for two minutes each. Lightly knead the inside of the spealbone as the final touches of the treatment.

Suggested Regimen

a. The disease may aggravate if the child catches cold. So see to it that the room is kept warm to prevent the onslaught of wind-cold on the child.

b. Do not take the child to public places to avoid further complications by the contagion of infectious diseases.

c. Feed the child properly by introducing a rational diet. Strengthen its physique and improve the health of the child.

Asthma

Asthma is common among children as a form of respiratory disease. A child is exposed to it in all seasons of the year, in particular, during the cold season or when there is a sudden turn of bad weather. Before asthma strikes a child it may find nasal mucosa itching, running nose, sneeze and not feeling well all over the body as premonitory symptoms. Following this the child may experience a sudden choking sensation in the chest, difficulty in breathing and asthma, which either occur for a short time or over a long period. In serious cases the child suffers from parted lips and huddled shoulders. It cannot lie down easily. Sweating copiously, cool limbs and venous engorgement in the neck are other symptoms.

Massage Method One

1. Prone position
a. The parent rubs the patient horizontally on the medial side of the spealbone with the bottom of the palm for three minutes.

b. Point and knead Dazhui, Feishu and Geshu for one minute each with thumb.

c. With thumb, index and middle fingers lift up Jianjing on either side 10 times.

2. Supine position
a. Using the Renmai as the middle line the parent pushes from Tiantu to the entire chest with fingers of both hands on either side for 2 minutes. Rub the chest for one minute.

b. Press and knead with middle finger Tiantu and Danzhong for one minute each.

c. The parent rests his/her palm on Shenque and rubs clockwise for one minute with navel as centre. Rub counter clockwise in spiral fashion for one minute. Push left and right of belly 50 times to wind up the operation.

Massage Method Two

1. Commonly used manipulations

a. Cleanse Feijing 300 times and massage Neibagua 100 times. Press and knead Xiaohenwen in the palm 200 times.

b. Press and knead Tiantu 20 times. Knead Danzhong 100 times. Push Danzhong left and right 50 times each.

c. Press and knead Dingchuan and Tianshu for one minute each. Lift up Jianjing 10 times.

2. Additonal manipulations

a. Asthma caused by the accumulation of cold. The symptoms are wheezing sound in the throat, stuffiness in septum pectorale, expectoration with scanty and white phlegm, afraid of cold, no perspiration, pale face, either not thirsty or like to have hot drinks, urine long and clean, tongue pale red with thin and white coating. To treat the case push Sanguan 300 times, press and knead Hegu and Fengchi 10 times each and push the spealbone separately 100 times each.

b. Asthma due to heat. Cleanse Dachang 100 times, push Liufu 200 times and press and knead Fenglong for 2 minutes, in case the child suffers asthma belonging to this type and has the following symptoms: wheezing sound in throat, choking sensation in chest, fidgeting, expectoration of yellow phlegm, badly wanting cold drinks, dark urine, constipation, fever with red face, red tongue, and thin and yellow coated tongue. To treat the case cleanse Dachang 100 times and push Liufu 200 times.

c. Asthma due to debility. Massage the Pijing, Feijing and Shenjing 200 times each for tonifying purpose. Press and knead Guanyuan and Sanyinjiao for one minute each. Knead Pishu and Shenshu for two minutes each, in case the child suffers from asthma due to debility with the following symptoms: repeated occurrence of asthma in sustained manner, weak cough, low voice and short of breath—the more so when the child moves about, lips, nails and toe becoming purple, tongue light and coated tongue thin and white.

Suggested Regimen

a. The child should be kept warm to avoid catching cold. Strengthen the child's immune system against disease.

b. Avoid coming into contact with air that causes stimulation, such as dust which is an allergen.

c. Only lightly seasoned foods are to be taken by the child. Avoid greasy, sweet or spicy food.

Vomit

Vomit is a common disease of the digestive organ among children, with usual symptoms, such as vomiting after taking food (the contents thrown up by stomach through mouth are acid and very stinking), nausea, belching out wind from the stomach, abdominal fullness and distension, low spirit, pale face or face reddening to the ears, and no desire to eat.

Massage Method One

1. Commonly used manipulations

a. Let the child lie on its back. The parent pushes straight with thumb on Danzhong in the belly for 1-3 minutes.

b. The parent pushes from Zhongwan to the sides of the navel 30-50 times with the thumb of both hands.

c. The parent rubs the belly clockwise and counter clockwise for one minute each direction.

d. Press and knead Zusanli and Neiguan for one minute each with the tip of the thumb.

2. Additional manipulations

a. Vomit may be caused by excessive eating, in which case the child vomits with great frequency, a stinking and filthy mouth, the contents of vomited stuff show undigested milk-like substance, plenty of stinking stools, semi-liquid like, constipation, and aversion to food. Other symptoms are: abdominal distension. The patient feels better after vomit. There is a tendency to vomit stinking stuff. No desire to eat. The colour of tongue light and tongue coating thick and greasy. First, cleanse Pijing 100 times and knead Banmen 300 times. Second, cleanse Dachang 200 times and push Liufu 100 times. Third, press and knead Zhongwan with fingers for 1-3 minutes.

b. Vomit of the cold type develops slowly. The child vomits undigested food which is thin, sticky and odourless. The child is in low spirit. The face is pale. Cool limbs. Bellyache. The child seeks warmth. Borborygmus. Stool thin, in semi-liquid form, containing undigested food. Urination is clear and abundant. Tongue tasteless and coated tongue thin and white. The common method to deal with the case is to massage Pijing 300 times for tonifying purpose. Knead Banmen 300 times and Wailaogong 50 times. Push Sanguan 300 times. Press and knead Guanyuan for one minute. Rub with thumb the shoulder and back as well as the lumbosacral region horizontal wise till diathermancy.

c. What is described in traditional Chinese medical literature as of the heat vomiting type is characterised by instant vomit as soon as the patient eats anything. The vomited stuff is stinking or in yellow liquid. The body of the patient is warm. The mouth is dry. The lips are red. Fidgeting and restless. Epigastric distension and pain. Loose and stinking stools. Constipation. Little and dark urine. The tongue red. The coated tongue yellow. The common methods of massage in dealing with this type of vomit is: first, massage Pijing and Xiaochang 200 times each for tonifying purpose. Second, massage Dachang 200 times for cleansing purpose. Push Liufu 200 times. Third, push Xiaohengwen 100 times with the side of the thumb. Fourthly, press and knead Tianshu on both sides for one minute each. Five, push Xiaqijiegu 100 times.

d. Another described as of the deficiency-fire type has such symptoms as frequent dry vomit, dry throat and tongue, red lips, loss of appetite, red cheeks, feverish sensation in palms and soles, dry stool, dark urine, tip of tongue red, and coated tongue thin and dry. To treat this type of vomit you may perform the following: massage Tianheshui and Ganjing 200 times each for cleansing purpose. Massage Shenjing 300 times for tonifying purpose. Lastly, push Yongquan 300 times.

Massage Method Two

1. Commonly used manipulations

a. Let the child lie on its back. The parent kneads Zhong-wan for one minute with the middle finger.

b. He or she may place thumb of both hands on the hypochondriac region on both sides of the xiphoid process and push sideways for 1-3 minutes each.

c. Pinch and knead Neiguan for one minute.

d. Lift up and pinch the muscle part of Pishu and Weishu with thumb, index and middle fingers 15-20 times for each acupoint on the child who lies on its belly. Press and knead the specified points for one minute each with thumbs.

2. Additional manipulations

a. For child whose vomit is caused by wind-cold, press and knead Quchi and Hegu for one minute each. Push and knead Taiyang 50 times. Cleanse Feijing and Dachang 200 times each.

b. For child who has weak stomach and spleen and suffers mental fatigue, massage Pijing 300 times for tonifying purpose, knead Banmen 300 times, pinch spinal column 5-7 times, and press and knead Zusanli for 1-3 minutes.

c. To deal with over eating and having eaten rotten food, cleanse Weijing and Dachang 300 times each. Knead Banmen 100 times. Massage or Yun Neibagua 100 times and push Xiaqijiegu 100 times.

Massage Method Three

1. Commonly used manipulations

a. Let the child sit down or lie on its belly. Hold the head of the child with one hand. Push with index and middle fingers of the other hand from the midpoint of the hairline at the back of the neck to Dazhui 300 times.

b. Yun Neibagua 50-100 times with the thumb in sequential order.

2. Additional manipulations

For dyspepsia caused by improper diet or over eating, knead Banmen 300 times. Knead belly from upper to lower parts and conversely for 1-3 minutes each. In addressing sick child with deficiency of spleen, massage Pijing 300 times for tonifying purpose and knead Zusanli for 1-3 minutes. For child afflicted with humid heat, massage Tianheshui 200 times for cleansing purpose and push Jimen 50 times. For child who vomits due to cold push Sanguan 300 times and rub its back till the back is warm.

Suggested Regimen

a. Vomit can be caused by many factors. Vomit occurs frequently in acute infectious diseases, such as epidemic cerebrospinal meningitis and encephalitis B and acute belly diseases (intestinal obstruction and intussusception), which are precursors of vomit. The parent must differentiate the disease and find out the cause of the disease. He or she must not try to stop vomit, simply because he/she sees a child vomits. It will make things worse and aggravate vomit. Only the right sort of treatment can be applied.

b. During vomit the parent should put the head of the child on one side to prevent inhalation which may cause pneumonia.

c. During vomit do not feed the baby with milk, administer medicine to the child or move the child about at will.

d. See to it that the child has a proper diet—eating at fixed times with the right amount of food. Let the child take vitamins and protein. Do not let the child have too much fatty food. After weaning the intake of food should be increased.

e. If the baby is fed improperly or with too much milk or when air is sucked by the baby during feeding, the baby may vomit milk. This is not a symptom of disease.

f. Serious cases of vomit may lead to dyscrasia and metabolism disorder, in which case venous transfusion should be administered.

Hiccup

Hiccup is the circulation of vital energy in the wrong direction with loud sound caused by a sudden tightening of muscles below chest, happening repeatedly and abruptly. The patient is unable to stop hiccup by himself. The common symptoms are that a child may hiccup, continuously or at intervals. It affects the chewing of food or speech making. Breathing and sleep may be affected as well. Hiccup is often accompanied by mental fatigue, fidgeting and crying by the child.

Massage Method One

1. Commonly used manipulations

a. Let the sick child lie on its back. The parent presses and kneads Tiantu and Danzhong with thumb for one minute each.

b. Let the child lie on its back. Knead and rub Zhongwan clockwise for five minutes with the palm of the hand.

c. Let the child lie on its belly. Press and knead Geshu, Weishu and Dachangshu for one minute each with thumb.

d. Rub the back of the child with palm till diathermancy.

2. Additional manipulations

a. The child may suffer from stomach excessive cold characterised by long and deep hiccups with feelings of discomfort in the gastral cavity. Hiccups are reduced due to heat but aggravate due to cold. The child takes less food. It does not feel thirsty. The tongue is light in colour. The tongue coating thin and pale. Under such circumstances the parent should push Sanguan 300 times. Press and knead Qihai and Zusanli for one minute each.

b. A child may suffer from stomach excessive heat type of hiccups making loud noises, stinking mouth and feeling thirsty. The child likes cold drinks. Scanty and dark urine or constipation. The tongue is red and tongue coating yellow. The parent may cleanse Weijing and push Liufu 300 times each. An additional measure is to press and knead Zusanli for two minutes.

c. Another type may be due to indigestion with short, frequent and loud hiccups, aversion to food, abdominal distension and fullness, and vomiting rotten and acid stuff. The tongue coating is thick and greasy. To deal with this type of hiccup the parent should massage Pijing 200 times for tonifying purpose and another 200 times for cleansing purpose. Dachang should be massaged 200 times for cleansing purpose and Banmen kneaded 50 times. Furthermore pinch Sifeng 10 times. Press and knead Zusanli for one minute.

d. The fourth type is due to obstruction of the circulation of vital energy or qi depression. There are repeated hiccups, abdominal distension and fullness. Hiccup occurs when the child is in poor spirit and alleviates when it is in a good mood. There may be nausea and bitter feeling in the mouth. The child eats less food than usual. The tongue coating is thin and pale. The parent should adopt the commonly used method of pushing straight Danzhong 100 times. Push the upper and lower parts of the belly 20 times each. Press and knead Neiguan and Zusanli for one minute each.

e. To deal with hiccups caused by deficiency of positive qi elements—characterised by low and deep hiccups, shortness of breath, pale face, cold limbs, reduced diet and mental fatigue, the colour of tongue pale and the coating thin and white—the parent should rub the navel for 5 minutes, press and knead Qihai for one minute, press and knead Pishu, Weishu and Shenshu for one minute each.

Massage Method Two

a. Let the sick child lie on its back. The parent rubs the navel clockwise for 5-10 minutes with palm.

b. Let the child lie on its back. The parent presses and-pressurises Zanzhu for 5-8 minutes with thumbs lightly at first and heavily afterwards.

c. Press and knead Neiguan on two sides for one minute each.

Massage Method Three

a. Let the child lie on its back. The parent presses Tianding on two sides for two minutes with the breadth of the middle fingers.

b. Let the child lie on its back. The parent uses thumb to press and knead Danzhong and Zusanli for two minutes each.

Suggested Regimen

a. Introduce good eating habit by avoiding excessive eating or drinking. During massage treatment the child is not allowed to take cold drinks, acid or hot food.

b. Keep the child warm.

c. The parent exerts some strength in massaging the child —lightly at first and then heavily. Excessive force should be avoided. The child should be able to receive the heavy massage. Stop the massage when the child can stand it no longer.

Anorexia

Anorexia means a child does not show any inclination to eat when food is presented to it. The child has a jaded appetite. It may even reject food altogether. This goes on for a long time. There are no sumptoms such as cold due to external factors or internal injuries. In recent years anorexia has become rather common, in particular, among children in cities. Occurrence is more common in families with only one child. Anorexia has the highest frequency in occurrence among 1-6-year-olds. The symptoms of anorexia are: no inclination to eat anything or the child no longer relishes any food. The face is pale, lacking in glossiness. The body is lean or slightly so. The mental condition of the child, however, is normal. Urination and bowel movements are basically normal.

Massage Method

1. Commonly used manipulations

a. Press and knead Zhongwan and Tianshu for one minute each.

b. Rub the abdomen clockwise and counter clockwise for three minutes.

c. Massage the belly from upper part to lower part 100 times. Press and knead Zusanli for one minute.

d. Pinch the spinal column repeatedly 10-15 times.

2. Additional manipulations

A. Anorexia caused by dysfunction of the spleen in transport. The child is pale without glossiness. Jaded appetite or tastelessness. The child refuses to take food. When the child eats excessively or is forced to take anything, the child feels ill in the stomach and wants to vomit. There is abdominal distension or fullness. The child becomes lean but there is nothing abnormal about its mental condition. Both urination and bowel movements are basically normal. Tongue coating is pale or thin, and not greasy.

a. To deal with this type of anorexia the parent should massage Pijing for tonifying purpose and knead Banmen 300 times each.

b. Yun Neibagua acupoint in sequential order 100 times. Press and knead Pishu and Weishu for one minute each.

B. Anorexia caused by stomach-Yin deficiency. Commonly seen symptoms are dry mouth and frequent drinking, jaded appetite, skin dry and without glossiness, stool hard and dry, and tongue uncoated and smooth. Sometimes the child may have uncoated and red tongue with scanty saliva. The commonly used manipulations for this type of anorexia are:

a. Massage Shenshui 300 times for tonifying purpose and knead Yongquan 100 times.

b. Press and knead Weishu for one minute.

Suggested Regimen

a. Readjustment should be introduced to the diet according to the principles of science. This is an important means to prevent anorexia. Dietary bias or partiality for a particular kind of food should be rooted out. Nibbling between meals and eating of candies should be stopped. Regular meals should be taken at fixed hours of the day.

b. Avoid mental stimulation. The child should lead a regular life.

c. In case anorexia occurs as a result of other diseases, the child should be sent to hospital for examination and proper treatment.

Abdominal Distension

This refers to distension and fullness of the entire gastric cavity or below the cavity. The belly becomes unusually large. If you strike it the belly will produce a sound as if you are hitting a drum. Another symptom is that the child does not eat much food yet feels it has a full stomach. It emits smell of rotting and acid food from the stomach through the mouth. Nausea and vomiting are features of this kind of disease.

Massage Method One

1. Commonly used manipulations
a. Let the child lie on its back. Knead Danzhong with the tip of the middle finger. Push straight the same acupoint with the bottom of the thumb 50 times. Push the upper and lower part of the belly 30 times.

b. Rub Zhongwan of the child, who lies on its back in bed for five minutes. Press and knead Shuifen for one minute.

c. Press and knead Zusanli for two minutes.

2. Additional manipulations
A. The first is described as of the indigestion type. The symptoms are distension and fullness of abdomen or gastric cavity, emitting smell of rotting and acid food from the stomach through the mouth, nausea, vomit, constipation, and bellyache. The child cannot stand any pressing of the belly by the parent. Tongue coating is greasy and thick.

a. Knead Banmen 50 times and massage Dachang 200 times for cleansing the large intestine.

b. Press and knead Tianshu for two minutes.

B. The second is known as obstruction of phlegm type. The symptoms are abdominal distension and fullness, fatigue and weariness or coughing up thick phlegm, and thick and greasy tongue coating.

a. Push Liufu 300 times.

b. Press and knead Fenglong 50 times and Pishu for one minute.

C. The third is known as deficiency of spleen type, characterised by distension and fullness of abdomen, and jaded appetite. The child seeks warmth and likes to be pressed. Other symptoms are shortness of breath, fatigue, semi-liquid stool, cool limbs, tongue pale, and thin and white tongue coating.

a. Massage Pijing 300 times and Dachang 100 times for tonifying purpose. Knead Banmen 50 times.

b. Press and knead Pishu and Weishu for one minute each.

c. Pinch and lift up the spinal column 5-10 times.

Massage Method Two

a. Let the child lie on its back. Yun Neibagua 100 times with thumb. Push Banmen 200 times.

b. Let the child lie in the same position. Rub Zhongwan for five minutes clockwise, using Dayuji. Push the upper and lower part of the belly 50 times.

c. Press and knead Tianshu, Pishu and Zusanli for one minute each.

Suggested Regimen

a.Distension of the abdomen is a common phenomena and sign of disease of the digestive system. Be careful to find out the cause of sickness. Address the problem properly according to the condition of illness.

b. Feed the child in a rational way. Cultivate a good eating habit.

c. Lead a well regulated life. Avoid stimulation caused by cold.

Abdominal Pain

This refers to pain below the gastric cavity and above the pubic or side bone, a common occurrence in child diseases. Clinical experiences tell us that pain may occur around the navel in the lower abdomen. Pain may be of different type—cold pain, burning pain, dull pain, colic pain, pain with distension, and prickling pain. The pain is often accompanied by lean body, pale face, crying, fidgeting and restlessness.

Massage Method One

1. Commonly used manipulations

a. Press and knead Zhongwan for one minute with index and middle fingers.

b. Pinch and lift up the muscular parts around Pishu, Weishu and Zhiyang on the back 20 times each.

c. Press and knead Zusanli and Neiguan for one minute each.

d. Rub the abdomen clockwise and counter clockwise for three minutes each.

2. Additional manipulations

a. Bellyache caused by cold factors has such syndromes as rather acute pain in the abdomen, crying, restlessness, preference for warmth (pain decreases when the child is warm), pale face, cool limbs; semi-liquid stool, dull urination, tongue pale, and tongue coating white. Knead Yiwofeng 50 times, push Sanguan 200 times, knead Wailaogong 50 times and pinch Dujiao five times.

b. In the case of pain caused by deficiency cold, the symptoms are: occasional or unending dull pain in the abdomen; the belly likes to be warm and there is an inclination to have the belly pressed; cool limbs, semi-liquid stool, leanness of body, tongue pale and tongue coating white. The commonly used manipulations are: massage Pijing 300 times for tonifying purpose. Knead Banmen 50 times. Press and knead Guanyuan and Mingmen for one minute each.

c. Pain caused by indigestion has the following symptoms: abdominal distension and pain; the child refuses to be pressed; disinclination to be fed with milk; and inclination to vomit rotten or acid stuff. There is pain and inclination to purge the bowels. The pain lessens after purgation. The tongue coating becomes thick and greasy. The commonly used manipulations to deal with the case are: cleanse Dachang and push Liufu 100 times each. Knead Banmen 50 times. Press Tianshu 50 times.

d. Periodic abdominal pain is caused by enterositosis around the navel, which occurs at times and then stops. The child has a strong desire to eat but its face is pale and the body is emaciated. The child does not sleep well or grinds teeth in sleep. On examination the stool reveals deposits of eggs of parasitic worms. The tongue pale, and tongue coating white. The commonly used manipulations to deal with this kind of pain include: cleansing the spleen acupoint for tonifying purpose 100 times. Cleanse Dachang 200 times, followed by lifting up Dujiao five times.

Massage Method Two

a. Let the child lie on its back. The parent points Zhong-wan with the thumb of the left hand. The thumb of the right hand pinches Sanyinjiao on both sides. The whole process takes 5 minutes.

b. Ths child lies on its back. Rub the navel counterclock-wise for five minutes. Lift up Dujiao three times.

c. Let the child lie on its back. Press and knead Pishu and Weishu for one minute each. Rub the back of the child till diathermancy.

Suggested Regimen

a. Abdominal pain is common among children. Its causes are rather complex. A thorough physical checkup should be made before massage is used. Diagnosis must be made early to prevent worsening of the disease.

b. The child should be kept warm. Care is taken to prevent the child from being attacked by external forces. A proper diet should be maintained. No excessive eating or drinking is allowed. Avoid intake of too much cold food. Do not eat any raw food.

c. When the child is pale with cold perspiration and has cool limbs, it should be sent to the hospital for treatment immediately.

Diarrhoea

Child diarrhoea is also known as indigestion—a disease of the alimentary tract caused by dysfunction of the spleen and stomach. The main symptoms are: frequent discharge of watery stools or stools in semi-liquid form, bellyache, nausea, fever, jaded appetite and emaciation.

Massage Method One

1. Commonly used manipulations:

a. Let the child lie on its back. Rub the abdomen counter-clockwise for five minutes with Dayuji.

b. Let the child lie on its belly. Push Qijiegu 300 times from bottom to top with thumb.

c. Press and knead Pishu, Weishu and Dachangshu for one minute each.

2. Additional manipulations

a. Diarrhoea among children is referred to as indigestion. If case history reveals indigestion during a recent period, the stool may be semi-liquid mixed with food relics, emanating a bad smell. The child feels nausea. It may vomit. There are halitosis and abdominal distension. The child cries and feels ill at ease before bowel movement. The tongue coating is thick and greasy. To deal with this case the common mani-pulation is: Cleanse Dachang 300 times and knead Banmen 200 times. Press and knead Tianshu (on both sides) and Zusanli for one minute each.

b. The second case is effusion characterised by urgent calls of dark, stinking stool with mucosa accompanied by bellyache. The mouth is thirsty and hot. Sometimes the child has no desire to drink anything in spite of thirst. The anus is warm. Scanty urination. Tongue becomes red. Tongue coating is greasy and yellow. To treat this case cleanse Pijing and Dachang 200 times each. Cleanse Xiaochang 100 times. Push Sanguan 100 times. Push Liufu 200 times. Press and knead Tianshu for two minutes.

c. The third case is diarrhoea of the cold type. There are light, thin and bubbling stools with slight or no bad smell, bellyache and borborygmus. The child has an aversion to cold and is afflicted with fever plus nasal discharge. The mouth is not thirsty. The tongue coating is white and greasy. The common manipulations to deal with this case are to massage Pijing 200 times for tonifying purpose, push Sanguan 100 times, knead Yuwei 300 times, and press and knead Zusanli for three minutes.

d. Diarrhoea due to spleen deficiency. The disease may last over a long period with little prospect of recovery. Diarrhoea may occur only intermittently but recurs many times. The stool is thin and liquid-like, containing undigested food relics. The face of the child is pale. The child is stricken by mental fatigue and depression. The tongue is tasteless and its coating thin and greasy. The commonly used manipulations are to cleanse Pijing and massage Dachang for tonifying purpose 300 times each, push Banmen 100 times, and press and knead Shenshu and Zusanli for two minutes each.

Massage Method Two

a. Let the child lie on its back. Push Pijing 300 times with ginger juice as media. Knead Banmen 200 times. Push Dachang 100 times.

b. Use the thumb or index and middle fingers to push Sanguan till the skin is red.

c. Rub the belly with Xiaoyuji from Zhongwan to the

surrounding parts of Shenque till the skin is hot and the massagist himself feels hot in the hand.

d. Let the child lie on the belly. Push Qijiegu with thumb from the fourth lumbar vertebra to Changqiang till the skin is red. Knead Guiwei heavily 10 times.

e. Pinch Zusanli on two sides with thumb for two minutes.

Suggested Regimen

a. In the course of massage, care should be taken to feed the child with fixed amount of milk or food at fixed times of the day. Take care that the child eats no unclean stuff. Protect the belly so that it will not catch cold. After each bowel movement the anus should be washed with warm water. Change the diaper constantly.

b. Massage is an effective way to heal the disease. Other treatments can also be given. In contagious diseases antibiotics may be used alongside massage. In case of loss of body fluid or if the child succumbs to poison, venous transfusion should be used.

Constipation

Constipation means unable to excrete the contents of the bowels often enough or there is difficulty in excretion. The child may be irregular in bowels or lacks a regular habit to excrete at fixed times of the day. As a result there is condiational reflex in excretion. Constipation is sometimes caused by excessive eating or lack of restraint in diet, which leads to lack of nutrition. The usual symptoms are dyschesia, feeling discomfort in abdomen, choking sensation in the chest, distaste for food, bad temper, fidgeting and crying.

Massage Method One

a. Let the child lie on its back. Press and knead Zhongwan, Tianshu and Zusanli for one minute each with the thumb.

b. Place the child in the same position. Press and rub Danzhong downward to Guanyuan below the navel 10 times, using the bottom of the palm. Alternate with the hands as the massagist manipulates with considerable force. Rub repeatedly along the regions of the colon ascendens, transversum, and descendens for five minutes. The massage should be conducted lightly, quickly and softly in shallow as well as deep parts. For colon transversum heavy pressure should be exerted. For colon descendens the pressure should be slight.

c. The child should lie on its belly. Push Xiaqijiegu downward 500 times with the thumb. Knead Guiwei for one minute.

Massage Method Two

1. Commonly used manipulations

a. Let the child lie on its back. Rub Zhongwan clockwise for five minutes. Press and knead Tianshu on both sides for three minutes.

b. Let the child lie on its belly. Push Qijiegu from top to bottom 400 times. Press and knead Pishu and Dachangshu for one minute each.

2. Additional manipulations

a. The first type has astriction characterised by dry stool, fullness of belly and pain, halitosis, vomiting gas, red face, fever, scanty and yellow urine, red tongue, and yellow tongue coating. The common manipulation is to cleanse Dachang and push Liufu 300 times each. Pinch and knead Zusanli for two minutes.

b. The second is described as constipation of the deficiency type, characterised by soft stool and impeded movement of bowels, mental fatigue, and lacking in strength, pale face, pale lips, tasteless tongue, and thin and white tongue coating. The common manipulation to deal with this case is to massage Pijing and Shenjing 300 times each for tonifying purpose and push Sanguan 300 times. Pinch and knead Zusanli for three minutes. Pinch and lift up the spinal column 5-10 times.

Suggested Regimen

a. The massagist should correct the life style of the child, such as changing improper dietary habit, eating corn or millet plus vegetables instead of wheat and rice. Form the habit of excreting at fixed times of the day. Take proper rest and end stresses and strains.

b. After massage if the child still suffers from constipation, use enema. Massage the parts as described.

Deficiency of Vitamin A

Deficiency in vitamins leads to skin and eye diseases. This kind of disease occurs frequently among some children, particularly infants. The symptoms are: dry skin is detected at first. The skin becomes scaly as small hard dry areas fall off in tiny pieces, more noticeably in parts of limbs which stretch or bend, and on shoulders. The hair becomes dry, lacking in glossiness. There may be loss of hair. The finger nails lack glossiness,too. Some children cannot see properly at night. Night blindness follows. Some children have fewer tears than usual. There are silver grains like bubbles in the white of the eye, known as conjunctiva spots. In serious cases the cornea may soften or perforate, which leads to blindness.

Massage Method One

1. Commonly used manipulations

a. Let the child lie on its back. Knead the abdomen clockwise with the palm of the hand for 2-5 minutes.

b. Press and knead Jingming, Zanzhu, Yangbai, Sibai and Tongziliao for 30 seconds to one minute each. Mop or daub the eye socket 10-15 times.

c. Grip and knead Xuehai 10-15 times.

d. Press and knead Fengchi and Zusanli for one minute each.

e. Let the child lie on its belly. Press and knead Ganshu, Pishu, Weishu and Shenshu for 30 seconds each.

2. Additional manipulations

a. The first case is where the spleen and stomach suffer deficiency, characterised by blurred eyesight at night, feeling dry in the eye and eyes blinking rapidly. The child likes to be in the dark and shies away from light. The skin of the entire body becomes dry and the face pale. The body becomes thin. Jaded appetite. Distension and fullness of abdomen. Semi-liquid stool. Tongue becoming tasteless and tongue coating white. The common manipulation to address this sickness is: massage Pijing 300 times for tonifying purpose. Knead Banmen 300 times. Push Sanguan 100 times. Press and knead Zhongwan and Tianshu for one minute each. Rub horizontally with palm the shoulder, back, hip and sacrum till the parts become warm.

b. Yin-deficiency in the liver, with symptoms, such as dry eyes, shying away from light, shedding tears, blurred eye vision at night, dry skin all over the body, dry throat and thirst, red cheeks, perspiration at night, warm sensation from fingers to toes, dry and hard stools, the tongue becoming red, and tongue coating thin. The common manipulation to deal with this type of disease is to massage Ganjing 300 times and Shenjing 100 times for tonifying purpose. Let the child lie on the back. Place thumbs of both hands on the hypochondriac region on both sides of the xiphoid process and push sideways 10-15 times. Rub Yongquan 300 times.

Massage Method Two

a. Let the child lie on its back. Push from Yintang to the front hairline with thumbs by turns 10-15 times. Press and knead Baihui for one minute.

b. Rub from Yintang to Taiyang 10-15 times with thumbs. Press and knead Taiyang for one minute.

c. Knead Jingming and Sibai for one minute each.

d. Hold the thumb apart from the other four fingers. Knead the muscle of limbs for 2-5 minutes.

e. Let the child lie on its back. Press and knead Ganshu, Pishuu, Weishu and Shenshu for one minute each with fingers.

Suggested Regimen

a. Feed the child with food rich in vitamin A regularly,

such as liver (from pig or sheep), egg yolk, carrot and spinach. Feed the child with fruits and dried almond to replenish carotene.

b. Feed the child with cod liver oil and inject vitamin AD according to prescription given by the doctor.

c. In dealing with consumptive diseases, consult with the doctor quickly and replenish the child with vitamin A.

Frequent urination

Frequent urination indicates more than usual amount of urine excreted with a sense of urgency but no feeling of pain. However, children under two years of age, may have frequent urination. This does not necessarily mean they are sick. The common symptoms of frequent urination are: the child may want to urinate perhaps over 10 times a day. The urine is scanty. The face looks pale. The limbs are cool. Dry mouth and thirst. There is mental fatigue or exhaustion.

Massage Method One

1. Commonly used manipulations

a. Massage Pijing 300 times and Shenjing 200 times for tonifying purpose.

b. Massage Xiaochangjing 200 times for the same purpose.

c. Let the child lie on its back. Touch Dantian with the bottom of the palm, massaging spiralling fashion clockwise for 2-5 minutes.

d. Let the child lie on its belly. Press and knead Shenshu

and Pangguangshu for one minute each.

e. Press and knead Sanyinjiao for 1-3 minutes.

2. Additional manipulations

a. Urinating frequently or in dribbling style belonging to the Qi-deficiency type is characterised by white and clean urine, pale face, cool limbs, cool belly, little talk by the child, dementia, tasteless tongue and thin and white tongue coating. The common manipulation is to massage Feijing 300 times for tonifying purpose. Pinch spinal column 5-10 times. Press and knead both sides of Pishu for one minute each. Press and knead Baihui for one minute. Rub the hip and back for one minute.

b. Disease of the Yin-deficiency type of urination is characterised by frequent urination or urinary incontinence, dark urine, fever at night and thirst, warmth in palm of hands and bottom of foot, red cheeks, red tongue, and thin tongue coating. The common manipulation is as follows: press and knead Baihui for 1-3 minutes. Knead Errenshangma 50 times. Massage Shenjing 500 times for tonifying purpose. Pinch Yinlingquan 3-5 times.

Massage Method Two

a. Let the child sit down or lie on its back. Knead Baihui for 1-3 minutes with the thumb.

b. Knead Errenshangma 30-50 times.

c. Let the child lie on its back. Place Xiaoyuji on the lower abdomen. Press and knead the abdomen with Dantian as the centre clockwise for 2-5 minutes.

d. Press and knead Shenshu for three minutes. Rub horizontally till the belly becomes warm.

e. Rub the upper chest horizontally. Rub in a straight manner from the back to the hip and sacrum till they become warm.

f. Press and knead Zusanli and Sanyinjiao for one minute each.

g. Rub Yongquan 20 times.

Massage Method Three

a. Let the child lie on its back. Press and knead Qihai clockwise 20 times with the middle finger breath. Press and knead Zhongji for one minute.

b. Let the child lie on its belly. Pinch the spinal column 10-15 times.

c. Press and knead and rub the lower end of the sacrum with the bottom part of the palm till the part becomes warm.

d. Press and knead Yinlingquan and Sanyinjiao for one minute each with fingers.

Suggested Regimen

a. Care should be taken to see whether the urethral orifice is red or swollen and whether changes have occurred in routine urinary test. If so medication should be given to put an end to urinary tract infections.

b. Let the child stay in bed. There should be no excessive work or stimulation for the child. See to it that the child does not catch cold. Keep its skin clean. Wash the child with warm towel once every day.

c. Do not scare the child when it urinates. Otherwise there will be dysfunction of the cerebral cortex, which will lead to frequent urination or urinary incontinence.

d. To deal with frequent urination caused by deficiency in kidney qi, Chinese patent drug, such as Liuweidihuangwan, should be administered to the patient to enhance the curative efficiency of massage treatment.

Enuresis

Enuresis (bed wetting) refers to urination inadvertently in bed during sleep by children over three year of age. Clinical practice tells us that in light cases the child may wet once each night and in serious cases once or several times on one night. A child who suffers from bed wetting over a long period of time may find its face emaciated or in a state of mental depression and intellectual deterioration. It loses its sense of taste for food.

Massage Method One

1. Commonly used manipulations

a. Let the child lie on its back. Press and knead Qihai and Guanyuan counter clockwise for five minutes each with the palm of the hand. Press and knead Zhongji with thumb for one minute.

b. Steady the child with one hand. With the Xiaoyuji of the other hand push Qijiegu from bottom to top till partially warm.

c. Press and knead Taixi and Sanyinjiao for one minute each.

2. Additional manipulations

a. Enuresis of the kidney and qi deficiency type has the following symptoms: urination in sleep one, two or more times every night, dullness of expression and of mind, cool limbs, aversion to cold, weak limbs and hip, urination in light colour and in large quantity, pale tongue and thin and white tongue coating. Massage Shenjing 300 times for tonifying purpose; press and knead Shenshu and Mingmen for one minute each.

b. For enuresis of the lung qi deficiency type character-ised by urination during sleep, increased urination in the day with reduced amount each time, mental fatigue, getting rather thin and lean in body, loss of appetite, watery faeces, tongue tasteless, and tongue coating thin and white, massage Pijing and Feijing 300 times each for tonifying purpose, push San-guan 300 times and press and knead Pishu and Shenshu for one minute each.

c. To address enuresis of the Ganjing humid-heat type with urination in sleep, which is frequent, yellow and short, irascible temperament, red face, red tongue tip and red tongue border, and thin and yellow tongue coating, cleanse Ganjing and Xiaochang 300 times each, cleanse Tianheshui 100 times, and press and knead Ganshu, Xiaochangshu and Xinshu for one minute each.

Massage Method Two

Hold the child in the hands or let it lie on its back. Push Pijing and Sanguan 300 times each, using talcum powder as a massage medium. Hold the child by the small finger. Push Shenjing 300 times. Pinch the centre of the traverse crease in the second digital joint of the small finger 10 times. This location is called bed wetting point. Hold the back of the hand of the child and knead Wailaogong 300 times. Let the child lie on its back, knead Zhongwan for five minutes. Press and knead Sanyinjiao for two minutes.

Suggested Regimen

Give words of encouragement and inject confidence in the curability of bed wetting in the patient. Cultivate in the patient the habit of urination at night. Do not let the child become too exhausted during the day. See to it that the child maintains a proper diet and takes a suitable amount of exercise. Massage once a day on 5-10 occasions continuously. If the child no longer wets the bed, massage a few more times to consolidate the gain.

Nocturnal Crying

This refers to morbid night crying of children at intervals or continuously, lasting the whole night. During day the child is quiet. The disease is common among babies less than three months old.

Massage Method One

a. Let the child lie on its back. Rub the belly with Dayuji clockwise and counter clockwise respectively for one minute.

b. Let the child lie on its belly. Press and knead Pishu, Xinshu and Zhiyang on the back for one minute each.

c. Press and knead Shenmen, Zusanli and Sanyinjiao for one minute each.

Massage Method Two

1. Commonly used manipulations

a. Massage Pijing 200 times for tonifying purpose. Cleanse Xinjing and Ganjing 200 times each.

b. With the child lying on its back, rub the belly clockwise with the palm of the hand and knead the navel for three minutes each. Press and knead Zusanli for one minute.

2. Additional manipulations

a. For Pi deficiency type with weak night cry, bellyache (during which the child likes to have its belly pressed by someone), cool limbs, eating less food and semi-liquid stool plus pale face, pale lips and tongue, and white and thin tongue coating, massage Banmen 300 times and push Sanguan 50 times. Pinch and knead Sihengwen 10 times. Rub Zhongwan for three minutes.

b. For internal heat type with loud night cry, red face and eyes, vexation, fear of bright light, dry stools, yellow urine, red tongue tip, and white tongue coating, cleanse Tianheshui and push Liufu 200 times each. Cleanse Xiaochang 300 times. Use the method known as "dredging the moon from under the water" 30 times.

c. For panicky type with crying at night bitterly, pale face, anxiety, sleeping fitfully, and thick tongue coating: Press and knead Shenmen and Baihui for one minute each. Knead Xiaotianxin 100 times. Pinch Weiling five times. Pinch Xinjing and Ganjing 50 times each.

d. To address night cry caused by indigestion, with symptoms such as crying and fidgeting, aversion to food, vomiting rotten and acid stuff, distension and fullness of the abdomen, stinking stool and thick and greasy tongue coating, knead Banmen and massage or Yun Neibagua 100 times each, cleanse Dachang 300 times, and knead Zhongwan for three minutes.

Suggested Regimen

Night cry should be dealt with by first finding out its causes, which may be hunger or excessive heat. Fever and rickets should be duly treated. Secondly, cultivate a good habit of going to sleep at regular times. The child should be adequately and suitably dressed in warm garment. Do not let the child catch cold. Finally the child should be fed with milk or food according to schedule and in fixed quantity to avoid indigestion.

Somniloquy

Somniloquy refers to a child frequently talking in sleep, accompanied by crying and restlessness. Sometimes sleep talking takes place a few days in a row, lasting even a month. The child behaves well in the day, though rather fatigued, weak and jaded in appetite.

Massage Method One

1. Commonly used manipulations
a. Let the child lie on its back. Rub your hands warm. Knead and rub the belly alternately, using the navel as the centre for 2-5 minutes.

b. Using fingers to massage Shenmen, Zusanli and Sanyinjiao for 1-3 minutes each.

c. With the child lying on its belly, the massagist rubs the back horizontally with palm till diathermancy.

d. Press and knead Xinshu, Jueyinshu, Pishu and Shenshu for 30 seconds to one minute each.

2. Additional manipulations
a. Sleep talking due to dysfunction of the spleen and stomach, has such symptoms as, fidgeting, distension and

fullness of the abdomen, jaded appetite, nausea, thin stool, tasteless tongue and greasy tongue coating. This can be healed by the following manipulations: Use two thumbs to press Zhongwan, pushing straight from middle to lower belly 5-10 times on the child who lies on its back. Cleanse and nourish Pijing 100 times each; Knead Banmen 200 times; Pinch Sifeng 5-10 times and pinch the spinal column 3-5 times.

b. Sleep talking due to excessive heat in Xinjing has such symptoms as, panicky shouts, restlessness, cries, red face and eyes, constipation, scanty and dark urine, red tongue tip, and thin and yellow tongue coating. To heal this type of illness the manipulations used include the following: Cleanse Xinjing 300 times and Xiaochang 100 times; Cleanse Dachang 100 times and push Liufu 100 times; Push and rub Yongquan 300 times and push Qijiegu downward 100 times.

c. Sleep talking may be of the violent panicky type with waking up suddenly at night in fear, seeking shelter in the embrace of the mother, light red tongue, and thin and white tongue coating. To address the problem cleanse Xinjing, Ganjing and Feijing 100 times each, and knead Zongjin 100 times. With the palm of hand rub shoulder, back, hip and sacrum till diathermancy.

Massage Method Two

a. Let the child lie on its back. The parent stands before the child, pushing and moping Yintang to the hairline with thumb of both hands 10-15 times. Press and knead Baihui for one minute.

b. With thumb of both hands massage from the centre of the forehead sideways to Taiyang 10-15 times. Press and knead the same acupoint for one minute.

c. The child lies on its back or is placed in a seating position. The parent bends fingers slightly. Exerting strength with the breadth of fingers, the parent grips and kneads the top of the head at the front to the top of the head at the back —repeatedly for 2-5 minutes.

d. The child lies on its back. The parent points at Qizhong with the palm and gives a shock treatment to the belly for one minute.

e. Press and knead Neiguan, Shenmen and Sanyinjiao for one minute each.

f. Let the child lie on its belly. The parent kneads the muscular parts by the spinal column from top to bottom with the bottom of the palm for 1-3 minutes. Press and knead sides of shanks for 30 seconds each.

Suggested Regimen

Massage stabilises the passion of the sick child and improves the condition of its sleep. The parent must not threaten the child by using rude language or corporal punishment. The food given to the child should be lightly seasoned and not too greasy, of the nutritious kind, and not hot or pungent. After one week of massage, if the disease is not cured, the child should be sent to hospital for treatment.

Convulsions

Convulsions are acute diseases common among children, characterised by jerks or spasm accompanied by delirium.

The popular Chinese term for the illness is chou feng or convulsive seizures. The symptoms include obnubilation, clenched teeth, spasm in limbs and convulsions.

Massage Method

Acute convulsions:

1. Commonly used manipulations

a. Pinch the philtrum or the vertical groove in the median line of the upper lip and Shixuan. Lift up Hegu and Taichong alternately till the child regains consciousness.

b. Grip Chengshan, Baichong and Quchi by turns till convulsions cease.

c. Cleanse Xinjing, Feijing and Ganjing 300 times each.

d. Let the child lie on its belly. Push the spinal column 50-100 times with the bottom part of the palm.

e. Press and knead Fenglong for 2-5 minutes.

2. Additional manipulations

a. Convulsions can be caused by cold. A child catching a slight cold may have symptoms, such as fever, cough, running nose, red throat, rigid limbs, eyes looking upward, clenched teeth, and thin and yellow tongue coating. In serious cases the child may have high temperature, very serious convulsions, red tongue and dry tongue coating. The common manipulation to deal with this type of convulsions is as follows: Cleanse Tianheshui 400 times and push Liufu 300 times. Knead Wailaogong 100 times. Press and knead Dazhui for one minute and push Yongquan 300 times.

b. Convulsions under excessive summer heat due to external factors are characterised by fever without sweat, headache, stiff neck, drowsiness and fidgeting by turns, spasm, thirst and constipation. In more serious cases the fever may last a sustained period, with repeated spasm and loss of consciousness. The common manipulation to deal with this kind of disease is to cleanse Tianheshui 500 times, push Liufu and Yongquan 600 times each, press and knead Dazhui for two minutes.

c. The humidity-heat poisonous type occurs in summer and autumn. The child may suddenly be seized by high fever, repeated spasm, fidgeting and delirium, thin and stinking stools mixed with purulent blood, red tongue, and yellow and greasy tongue coating. To treat this illness cleanse Xinjing 100 times. Cleanse Dachang and Xiaochang 400 times each, push Liufu 300 times, and press and knead Tianshu for 1-3 minutes.

d. The indigestion type is symtomised by abdominal distension and bellyache, nausea, vomit, fever, constipation, shortness of breath, eyes always looking straight, delirium and spasm, and the coated tongue thick and greasy. The common manipulation to deal with the case is to cleanse Dachang 400 times; knead Banmen 100 times; press and knead Zhongwan and Zusanli for 1-3 minutes each and massage Neibagua 300 times.

e. The panicky type, characterised by alarm, restlessness, pale face, unable to sleep, crying in sleep, eyes not steady and spasm in four limbs. The common manipulation to deal with the case is to press and knead Baihui for 1-3 minutes, knead Wailaogong and Xiaotianxin 100 times each and press and knead Shenmen for one minute.

Recurrent convulsions:

1. Commonly used manipulations

a. Massage Pijing and Shenjing 300 times for tonifying purpose. Cleanse Ganjing 300 times.

b. Rub Zhongwan for 2-5 minutes.

c. Push Sanguan 100 times.

d. Press and knead Baihui and Zusanli for one minute each.

e. Pinch the spinal column 5-10 times.

2. Additional manipulations

a. Recurrent convulsions described as of the weakness of spleen and stomach type are characterised by eyes open during sleep, pale and sallow face, jaded appetite, thin or watery stools, cool limbs, recurrent convulsions but with no vigorous convulsive movement, tasteless tongue and white tongue coating. To deal with the case massage Pijing 400 times for tonifying purpose. Knead Banmen 300 times. Press and knead Pishu, Weishu and Dachangshu for one minute each. Knead the navel 20 times and press Tianshu 10 times.

b. Recurrent convulsions of the insufficiency of both spleen and kidney type, are characterised by psychopathy, dark face, cool limbs, delirium, eyes open during sleep, semi-liquid stool, clear and abundant urine, wriggling limbs, tasteless tongue, and thin and white tongue coating. This can be cured by using the following manipulations: Rub Dazhui and Mingmen till they become warm. Massage Pijing 400 times and Shenjing 300 times for tonifying purpose. Press and knead Pishu, Shenshu and Taixi for one minute each.

c. Recurrent convulsions described as of the deficiency of liver-yin and kidney-yin type are characterised by lean body, low spirit, drowsy feeling, palm to sole becoming warm, shivering limbs, perspiration, dry stool, red tongue, and reduced saliva on tongue coating. To deal with the case the common manipulation is to push Yongquan 100 times and press and knead Ganshu and Shenshu for one minute each.

Suggested Regimen

a. In acute convulsions the disease occurs suddenly. Emergency measures are called for. As a first step massage the child. Send the child to hospital at once.

b. When convulsions occur take care that the child does not hurt its tongue due to clenching or teeth gritting. The child should be dressed in loose and comfortable clothing. Remove any secretions from the throat such as phlegm and keep the respiratory organ clean so that the child won't suffocate.

c. Do not try to pull the child's hands or feet forcibly during convulsion so that there won't be any after effects from convulsions.

d. Send the child to hospital immediately if complications develop into encephalitis B and epidemic cerebrospinal meningitis. If they do, massage can only be a supplementary step. Proper treatment should be given to the child by the doctor in the hospital.

Facial Paralysis

Facial paralysis is a disease indicated by obstructions of muscular movement due to nerve injury on the face. The Chinese term for this disease is: miantan or kouyewanxia, meaning facioplegia or mouth and eyes crooked or askew. The disease occurs suddenly. The child may discover that it cannot close its eye on one side and the mouth is crooked to one side as well when it wakes up one morning. The child cannot cleanse its mouth. The face is swollen or impeded. Usually there is pain below the ear or in the mastoid process. The expressions on the afflicted face disappear. The groove below nose and above upper lip becomes shallow. The child speaks indistinctly and slobbers. Saliva drops from the mouth. In eating the child leaves food in the teeth on the afflicted part of the face. The sense of taste may decline while hearing may be over sensitive.

Massage Method One

a. The child lies at its back or is placed in a seated position. The parent rubs the forehead to Taiyang on both sides with thumbs 15-30 times. This is followed by pressing and kneading the same acupoints for one minute each.

b. The child lies on its back with its head bent on the side of the unaffected side of the face. The parent rubs lightly with the bottom of the palm the side of the face suffering from paralysis till diathermancy.

c. Press and knead Yangbai, Sibai, Yingxiang, Dicang, Jiache and Xiaguan with the tip of the middle finger for 30 seconds to one minute each.

d. Press, knead and pluck Hegu vis-a-vis the affected and unaffected parts with the tip of the thumb for one minute each.

e. The child lies on its belly. The parent rubs the muscular parts lateral to the spinal column with palm till diathermancy.

f. The child is placed in a seated position. The parent lifts up the forehead with one hand, presses and kneads Fengchi with thumb and middle finger till a partial feeling of distension and pain is felt in the acupoint.

Massage Method Two

a. The child lies on its back. The parent presses and kneads both sides of the forehead with the breadth of the thumb for 1-3 minutes.

b. The child lies on its back, keeping the eyes shut as much as possible. The parent lightly kneads the surrounding part of the eyelid for 1-3 minutes with the breadth of the index finger. The parent must not touch eyes or injure the skin during manipulation.

c. The parent rubs own hands quickly till they are warm. Press the forehead of the child with the warm hand and rub the face counter clockwise and clockwise starting from the forehead, cheeks, ears, lower jaw and then from both cheeks back to the forehead 30 times each till the face is red and warm.

d. Press and knead Yingxiang for one minute with the index finger till there is a feeling of pain and distension in the acupoint.

e. The child is placed in a seated position. The parent presses Fengchi on both sides with thumbs, shaking the acupoint in a rhythmic manner, producing a marked sensation of fullness and pain in the acupoint. The manipulation lasts one minute.

f. Holding the earlobe with thumb and index finger, the parent kneads and pinches, lifting up in a ring-like manner till there is a sensation of pain in the earlobe. However there must not be any pain in the basal part (root of the ear). The entire ear becomes red and warm after the manipulation, which lasts 1-3 minutes.

Massage Method Three

a. The child lies on its back. Push Baihui with the thumb.

Push and knead Yintang first and then Jingming, Tongziliao, Taiyang, Jiache, Dicang, Yingxiang, Fengchi, Fengfu, Lianquan, Renzhong, and Hegu beside the stricken parts of the face for 5-10 minutes.

b. The child is placed in a seated position. The parent lightly lifts up and pinches the muscular parts of the affected side of the face tensely at first and relaxs afterwards for 5-10 times. The parent exerts force with the thumb, index and middle fingers during the operation.

c. The parent places the breadth of four fingers or Xiaoyuji on the affected side of the face and rubs lightly, till the face becomes warm.

Suggested Regimen

a. See to it that the child does not become over fatigued when it is receiving massage treatment. Take care that the child does not catch cold. Do not wash the face of the child with cold water.

b. Let the child do some exercise to increase its power of resistance to disease.

c. The use of heavy force should be avoided in manipulation by the massagist during the initial period.

d. Massage on affected and unaffected parts of the face can be undertaken by turns or simultaneously. The unaffected side needs only light manipulation whereas the affected side calls for heavy massage.

e. Older children should be taught to do self massage regularly to enhance efficacy of treatment in addition to receiving treatment from the parent.

Whooping Cough

Whooping cough is also known as pertussis, an acute infectious and epidemic disease in the respiratory organ caused by the hemophilus pertussis, which attacks children in all seasons of the year, particularly in winter and spring and among those under 5 years of age. Whooping cough can be very critical among younger children and lead to pneumonia on account of their tender age. The disease can last as long as three months. The Chinese call it hundred-day cough. The usual symptoms resemble cold with running nose, shedding tears, feeling hot in nose, red eyes, afraid to see bright light, sneeze, dry throat and fever. Gradually it develops into twitching cough, dry and itching throat. The attack occurs 10-20 times a day.

Massage Method One

1. Commonly used manipulations

a. The child lies on its back. The parent stands in front of the child's head, placing two palms on both sides of Tiantu and pushing along the intercostal region from the inside to the midaxillary line on the outside. Push from top to Rugen on the flat and high intercostal region. The massage lasts 1-5 minutes.

b. The child lies on its belly. Rub with the entire palm along the inside of the spealbone till diathermancy.

c. Press and knead Dazhui, Feishu and Dingchuan for one minute each.

d. Press, knead and pluck Zusanli and Fenglong for one minute each.

e. Knead the small traverse crease of the palm 200 times.

Cleanse Feijing 300 times.

2. Additional manipulations

a. Whooping cough of the wind-cold type with exterior syndrome of high fever, aversion to cold, headache and pain in the body but no persiration should be given the following treatment: push Sanguan 300 times, grip Fengchi and Hegu 10 times each, and rub the chest horizontally for one minute.

b. Whooping cough of the wind heat type with exterior syndrome of high fever, slight aversion to cold, little perspiration, red throat and face can be treated in the following way: cleanse Feijing and push Liufu 300 times each. Press and knead Quchi 30 times. Knead Hegu 10 times.

c. Whooping cough known as the serious phlegm-heat type is indicated by shortness of breath, cough, thick and sticky yellow phlegm, the mouth and nose heated up with qi and choking sensation in the breast. The common manipulation to deal with this type is to press and knead Fengchi, Quchi and Hegu for one minute each. Press Danzhong for one minute. Rub the sternal ribs for 1-5 minutes. Grip and knead the muscular parts beside the cervical vertebra with index and middle fingers and the thumb 5-10 times.

d. For cases with Qi deficiency in both spleen and lung indicated by weak coughing, fatigue, jaded appetite, whitish face and semi-liquid stool, the common manipulation is: massage Pijing and Feijing for tonifying purpose 300 times each. Press and knead Pishu, Feishu and Weishu for one minute each. Rub Zhongwan for three minutes. Pinch spinal column three times.

Massage Method Two

1. Commonly used manipulations

a. Let the child lie on its back. Place the index finger on

the middle finger. Point and knead Tiantu for one minute with the said fingers.

b. With the child lying on its back, squeeze and pinch the muscle in Danzhong with index and middle fingers and the thumb till part of the muscle becomes red.

c. Cleanse Feijing 300 times. Push Tianheshui 100 times. Push Liufu 200 times.

d. Press and knead Feishu 20 times. Pinch and knead Fenglong 10 times.

2. Additional manipulations

a. During initial period when whooping cough with exterior syndrome occurs push Zanzhu 10 times and Taiyang 10 times, grip Fengchi 10 times and Jianjing 3 times respectively.

b. To deal with spastic whooping cough knead the Yujijiao 300 times. Press and knead Yiwofeng 200 times. Massage or Yun Neibagua 100 times in the same direction.

c. In the convalescent period rub Zhongwan for five minutes. Press and knead Zusanli for one minute. Rub the back of the child horizontal-wise for one minute.

Massage Method Three

a. The child lies on its back. Grip and pinch Tiantu 50 times with index and middle fingers and the thumb.

b. The child lies on its belly. Press and knead Feishu on the back for 1-3 minutes with thumbs of both hands. Apply ginger juice to the back and hips alongside the spinal column and push with Xiaoyuji energetically up and down till diathermancy.

c. Press and knead Ceze, Fenglong, Hegu and Zusanli for one minute each.

d. Knead the small traverse crease in the palm 200 times.

Massage the Neibagua 100 times.

Suggested Regimen

a. Steps should be taken to give early diagnosis of whooping cough, which is an acute infectious respiratory disease. The child should be kept in isolation ward to prevent the spread of the disease.

b. Preventive measures must be taken, such as providing whooping cough bacterial vaccine. Avoid any contact with children afflicted with the disease. Do not take the child to public places when whooping cough is prevalent in winter.

c. See to it that the child is kept in healthy and quiet surroundings. Let the child be happy and do some exercise outdoor daily.

d. Let the child have more meals a day but less food each. After whooping cough feed the child to maintain its nutrition intake.

e. When a baby whooping coughs with spasm, it may easily lead to suffocation. Artificial respiration should be given and oxygen provided to help the child breathe.

f. When complication such as pneumonia develops the child should be given treatment at once to avoid aggravating the disease.

Dysentery

Dysentery is an infectious disease of the alimentary tract,

characterised by bellyache, tenesmus and dark stool with white thick blood. Bowel movements become very frequent but the patient is unable to empty the bowel. It is accompanied by aversion to cold, fever, loss of appetite, nausea, vomit and thin body.

Massage Method One

1. Commonly used manipulations

a. Let the child lie on its back. Rub Zhongwan clockwise with the palm of the hand for one minute.

b. Let the child lie on its back. The parent puts one palm on top of the other in an overlapping manner. He/she presses and pressurises lightly against the navel, shaking it for one minute. The parent lifts up the palms suddenly. The parent presses and relaxes in this way 5-10 times.

c. Let the child lie on its belly. Press and knead Pishu, Weishu and Dachangshu for one minute each.

d. Press and knead Tianshu and Zusanli for one minute each.

2. Additional manipulations

a. Dysentery described as of the humid-heat type is most common, characterised by bellyache, tenesmus, bloody stools, fever, thirst but no desire to drink, scanty and urgent urination, dementia, red tongue and yellowish and greasy tongue coating. To deal with this disease take the following measures: cleanse Dachang and push Liufu 300 times each; cleanse Xiaochang 200 times; push Xiaqijiegu 300 times; and press and knead Yanglingquan and Sanyinjiao 20 times each.

b. Dysentery of the damp-cold type is indicated by viscous, whitish, congealing stool, aversion to cold and wanting to be warm, cool and painful limbs, bellyache, borborygmus, taking less food than usual, mental fatigue, tasteless tongue, and white and greasy tongue coating. To heal the disease, massage Pijing 300 times and Dachang 100 times both for tonifying purpose. Press and knead Shangjuxu, Quchi and Hegu for one minute each.

c. Dysentery of the epidemic and poisonous type is indicated by high fever, thirst, headache, discharge of purulent, bloody stools, tenesmus, coma, red tongue and yellow tongue coating. The common manipulation to deal with this type of disease is to cleanse Weijing and Dachang 300 times, push Liufu 300 times and cleanse Tianheshui 300 times in the order stipulated. Pinch the philtrum, grip Hegu and pinch Shixuan till the child recovers consciousness.

d. Dysentery of the insufficiency-cold type is characterised by long affliction, dull pain in belly, insipid taste but not thirsty, taking in little food, mental fatigue, aversion to cold, cool limbs, tasteless tongue and thin and white tongue coating. The common manipulation to deal with this type of disease is to massage Pijing 300 times and Shenjing 200 times for tonifying purpose. Knead Dantian 100 times. Rub it with palm for three minutes. Press and knead Shenshu and Mingmen 20 times each.

e. Dysentery of the dormant type indicated by fitful excretion followed by a dormant period. Other symptoms include purulent, bloody stools, tenesmus, bellyache, reduced food intake, tiredness, aversion to cold, tasteless tongue and greasy tongue coating. The common manipulation to deal with the case is to massage Pijing 300 times and Dachang 100 times for tonifying purpose. Push Shangqijiegu 300 times. Press and knead Shangjuxu for one minute.

f. Dysentery of the tongue-tied type is indicated by red and white stool, tenesmus, dull pain in belly, aversion to food or drink, intake of food always followed by nausea and vomit, the tongue becoming tasteless and tongue coating greasy. The common manipulation to deal with this disease is: cleanse Xinjing and Ganjing 100 times each, massage Baigua 300 times, press and knead Weizhong and Chengshan for one minute each and rub the hip and sacrum till diathermancy.

Massage Method Two

a. Let the child lie on its back. Rub the belly below the navel with the palm of one hand clockwise and counter clockwise for 2-5 minutes.

b. Let the child lie on its belly. Push from the sacrum to the back with the bottom of the palm till diathermancy.

c. Press and knead Zusanli for three minutes. Press and knead Pishu, Weishu, Dachangshu and Tianshu for one minute each.

d. Push Tianheshui 500 times and Liufu 300 times in case the child has high fever. If the child is in a coma with convulsions, pinch the philtrum, Xiaotianxing and Shiwang by turns until the child gains consciousness. If the child has suffered from dysentery for a long period of time and is weak in constitution knead the antidiarrheal acupoint known as Zhili 10 times. Knead Errenshangma 30 times. Massage Pijing 300 times for tonifying purpose.

Massage Method Three

a. Let the child lie on its back. Press and knead Zhongwan, Tianshu and Zusanli for one minute each.

b. Let the child lie on its back. Knead the navel clockwise with the palm of the hand softly and quickly.

c. Let the child lie on its back. Rub the hypochondrium on both sides for 3-5 minutes with entire palm of both hands.

d. Let the child lie on its belly. Rub hands warm. Putting

the bottom part of the hand closely on both sides of the spinal column, push and rub from Shenshu to Dachangshu back and forth till diathermancy or radiant heat.

Suggested Regimen

a. The child should be in isolation during treatment till one week after the stool becomes normal. All utensils used by the child should be disinfected. Clothing and bed sheet should be washed constantly and kept clean. The massagist should wash hands diligently to prevent infection.

b. The room where the child stays should be nice, cool and quiet to provide the condition for the child to convalesce.

c. Let the child drink lots of beverages, preferably water containing sugar and salt or fruit juice. Fluid transport therapy should be undertaken for children suffering from serious dysentery.

d. Replenish the child with nutrition and vitamins. Do not give the child cold drinks or cold food to prevent undue wriggling movement of the stomach and intestines.

e. A close watch on the condition of sickness should be kept over the child. If sudden fidgeting and cool limbs occur call in the doctor at once for treatment.

Purulent Tympanitis

Purulent tympanitis is festering middle ear or tympanum caused by pyococcus. It falls into two categories: acute and chronic. It is a commonly seen disease among babies, characterised by crying for pain in the ear in the case of older children. In the case of younger ones cries are heard far more often, gripping the ear and shaking the head in pain. The babies often wake up in fear, crying. In serious cases high fever appears, accompanied by convulsions. These disappear, however, after the drumhead becomes perforated and pus occurs. As the disease continues over a long period of time it becomes chronic. Fluid formed by suppuration becomes a recurrent phenomenon. The drumhead is perforated. Hearing is affected or deteriorates. More often than not conductive deafness appears.

Massage Method One

1. Commonly used manipulations

a. Press and knead Yifeng behind the earlobe with thumb for 1-3 minutes.

b. Pluck Taixi on both sides with tip of the thumb 15 times each. Press and knead Taixi for one minute each.

c. Press and knead Fengchi for 1-3 minutes with thumb and middle finger.

d. Let the child lie on its belly. Push both sides of the spinal column with the bottom of the palm. The priority is Shenshu, which should be pushed for 1-3 minutes repeatedly.

2. Additional manipulations

a. Inflammation of the middle ear of the wind-heat type, occurring frequently in acute cases, is indicated in the initial stage by slight pain in the ear, which worsens as time goes on. The pain becomes prickly. The baby cries. It is stricken by fever sometimes. Other symptoms are: aversion to cold, headache, discomfort all over the body, red tongue, and thin and yellow tongue coating. The common manipulation is to cleanse Feijing and Tianheshui 300 times each.

Cleanse Dachang 100 times. Push Liufu 100 times. Press and knead Hegu and Quchi for one minute each. Rub Yongquan 100 times.

b. Humid-heat in the liver and kidney type occurs often in acute inflammation of the middle ear with pus flowing due to suppuration. It is seen among babies with chronic inflammation of the middle ear which occurs in an acute manner. It is characterised by pains in the ear, thick, stinking pus flowing continuously, accompanied by fever, constipation, yellow or red urine, tasteless tongue, and yellowish and greasy tongue coating. The common manipulation to heal the disease is to cleanse Ganjing and Tianheshui 300 times each. Knead Neilaogong 100 times. Cleanse Xiaochang 200 times. Press and knead Sanyinjiao for one minute. Push Xiaqijiegu 300 times.

c. Yin-insufficiency in liver and kidney type occurs often in chronic inflammation of the middle ear, with thin pus flowing in the ear intermittently. Other symptoms include weakened hearing, pale face, fatigue, tasteless tongue, and thin tongue coating. The common manipulation to deal with the disease is to massage Ganjing and Shenjing 200 times each for tonifying purpose. Push and rub Yongquan 50 times. Press and knead Sanyinjiao for one minute. Press and knead Ganshu and Shenshu for one minute each.

Massage Method Two

a. Cleanse Dachange 100 times. Push Liufu 100 times. Cleanse Tianheshui 200 times.

b. Cleanse Ganjing 100 times. Massage Shenjing 300 times for tonifying purpose. Knead Xiaotianxin 300 times.

c. Press and knead Fengchi, Waiguan and Sanyinjiao for one minute each.

d. Pinch Taichong on both sides for 15-20 seconds each.

e. Let the child lie on its belly. Rub the muscle of the shoulder, back, hip and sacrum from top to bottom with one palm repeatedly till diathermancy.

Suggested Regimen

a. Take active measures to prevent and cure infection of the upper respiratory tract and acute infectious diseases.

b. The child should not be in a lying position during feeding.

c. Let the child relax and rest. Activities should be curtailed. Do not move the baby about to reduce pain. After the drumhead is perforated place the child on the side of the afflicted ear so that the pus may flow out easily.

d. Intake of easily digestible food should be provided, such as liquid or semi-liquid food—rice soup, and soup consisting of well-cooked cereals, and milk.

e. Massage acts as a supplementary measure. Injection and medicine must be used to treat tympanitis. Consult with the doctor.

f. If the temperature continues to rise ever higher with strong headache, vomit, stiff neck and loss of consciousness in spite of massage, the child should be sent to hospital for treatment.

Nosebleed

Nosebleed (nasal hemorrhage) is sometimes called *binu*

(epistaxis) in Chinese, which refers to nosebleed due to rupture of blood vessel resulting in bleeding in the nasal cavity. It occurs rather often among children in all seasons of the year. The usual symptom is bleeding in one side of the nose, which hardly stops. In more serious cases blood comes out from the mouth or from the other side of the nose. Bleeding in profusion over a long time may result in pale face, cold sweat, quick but weak pulses and drop in blood pressure.

Massage Method One

1. Commonly used manipulations
a. The child should be placed in a sitting position or lie on its back. Pressurise against Yingxiang on both sides with the breadth of the thumb for 1-3 minutes each.

b. Pinch with force the philtrum or Renzhong with the tip of the thumb for 1-3 minutes.

c. Pinch Shangxin for one minute with index finger.

d. Press and knead Hegu on both sides for 1-3 minutes each with thumb.

2. Additional manipulations
a. Nosebleed of the type known as wind-heat in the lung is indicated by symptoms such as nosebleed, mucus of the nose containing blood, thirst, dry throat, cough with little phlegm, fever, aversion to wind, pain in head and body, red tongue and thin and yellowish tongue coating. The common manipulation to deal with this type is to cleanse Feijing and Tianheshui 300 times each, press and knead Dazhui and Quchi for one minute each, rub the back, hip and sacrum for 1-3 minutes.

b. Nosebleed of the stomach excessive heat type indicated by nasal cavity bleeding in profusion in red plus bleeding in the gum of the teeth, thirst, fidgeting, restlessness, halitosis, constipation, yellow or red urine, red tongue, and yellow tongue coating. The common manipulation to deal with the case is to cleanse Dachang and Weijing 300 times each, push Liufu 200 times, press and knead Zusanli on both sides for 1-3 minutes each, and push Xiaqijiegu 300 times.

c. Nosebleed of the liver fire-flaming type is characterised by nose bleeding intermittently, dizziness, hot temper, red face and eyes, red tongue, and yellow tongue coating. To heal the disease cleanse Xinjing 100 times and Feijing 200 times; rub Yongquan for 1-3 minutes with fingers; and press and knead Sanyinjiao and Taichong for one minute each.

d. Nosebleed of the insufficiency in qi-blood type is characterised by bleeding in faint red, fatigue, lacking in strength, dizziness, pain in hip and weak lower limbs, tasteless tongue, and thin and white tongue coating. To heal the disease massage Pijing 300 times for tonifying purpose. Knead Banmen 300 times. Rub Zhongwan for 2-5 minutes. Press and knead Pishu and Weishu for one minute each. Pinch the spinal column 5-7 times.

Massage Method Two

a. Place the child in a reclining or seating position. Pinch the nose with thumb and index finger. Let the child breathe with its mouth for 1-3 minutes.

b. Press Yingxiang on both sides of the nose with the tip of thumb and index finger. Pressing is followed by kneading for 1-2 minutes till there is pain and a sensation of expansion in parts of the acupoint.

c. Point at and pressurise against Fengchi with thumbs. Press it with force for one minute. Knead it 15-20 times.

Suggested Regimen

a. The parent should remain calm when he/she finds the child's nose bleeding. Sit the child up or place the child in a reclining position with head slightly bent forward. Place a basin before the child so that the blood may drop into the basin. Let the child relax. Take steps to stop bleeding.

b. Cool treatment should be given to the forehead or neck during or after bleeding. Use a towel and cold water for the purpose. Dip the towel in cold water once every two minutes.

c. Let the child eat vegetables, fruit and cool and appetising food. Do not give the child hot stuff, such as mutton, onion or ginger.

d. Cultivate a good healthy habit. Educate the child not to pick nose or do dangerous games to avoid injuring the nose.

e. During dry season let the child drink more water.

f. If bleeding occurs again and again, send the child to hospital.

Aphtha

Aphtha refers to parts of shallow surface in the mouth or tongue becoming ulcerated or festered, to which children of any age may succumb. It occurs more often among babies. The symptoms are: inside of lips and jaw, tongue, gum of teeth and the hard palate are affected by yellowish or white ulcers singly or in group. The borders of ulcers appear red. The surface has burning pain. There is slight halitosis. Saliva increases and becomes sticky. The child is restless and has a jaded appetite. The body is lean. There may be fever.

Massage Method One

1. Commonly used manipulations

a. Massage Shenjing 300 times for tonifying purpose and cleanse Tianheshui 200 times.

b. Cleanse Xiaochangjing 300 times and push Liufu 100 times.

c. Press and knead Hegu for 1-3 minutes with fingers.

d. Press and knead Zusanli for one minute each.

e. Push and rub Yongquan 30-50 times.

2. Additional manipulations

a. Aphtha of the type known as accumulation of heat in heart and spleen is characterised by red borders on the ulcerated mouth, burning pain, restlessness, halitosis and drooling, jaded appetite, constipation, scanty and dark urine, red tongue and yellow tongue coating. The common manipulation to deal with the case is to cleanse Xinjing 300 times and Dachang 200 times, rub from hip and back to sacrum 5-10 times and push Xiaqijiegu 300 times. The final steps to be taken are to leave a few drops of cold water on the palm of the child. Massage Shuidi beside the small finger. The Mingyue acupoint is at the tip of the middle finger when you clench your fist. Push the acupoint in spiral fashion. In so doing blow cold air into the acupoint 20 times. This is known as "dredging the moon out from under the water."

b. Aphtha of deficiency-fire type is indicated by irascibility, light red parts bordering ulcer, mental fatigue, lean body, red cheeks, dry mouth, thirst, slight halitosis, red tongue, and thin tongue coating. The common manipulation to deal with the case is: push and rub Yongquan 100 times. Rub Shenshu and Mingmen horizontal wise till diathermancy. Knead Sanyinjiao on both sides for one minute with fingers. Pinch Yinlingquan 10 times.

Massage Method Two

a. Cleanse Xinjing 300 times. Cleanse Tianheshui 200 times. Knead Zongjin 30 times.

b. Push Xiaohengwen 50-100 times.

c. Cleanse Xiaochang 100 times. Knead Xiaotianxin 50 times.

d. Rub Yongquan for 3-5 minutes.

e. Rub the muscle in hip, back and sacrum with the bottom of the palm till diathermancy.

f. Press and knead both Zusanli for one minute each.

Suggested Regimen

a. The child suffers terribly as aphtha occurs time and again. So care must be taken to nurse the child, who should not eat food that is too hot or too hard or too pungent. The child should only take liquid food.

b. Keep the mouth clean. Wash it with lukewarm water regularly.

c. In serious cases the child may run a high fever and get fidgety. Administer medicine and give injection to the child as scheduled. The child in high fever should be washed with alcohol as a physical means to bring down temperature. Use warm water to bathe the child. Administer medicine orally to the child to allay fever or kill pain.

Salivation

Salivation refers to flowing of saliva from mouth of the child unconsciously. It is known in Chinese as zhiyi or wet cheek or liu kou shui (saliva dribbling from the mouth), common among children under three years of age. However since a baby has a shallow mouth cavity and does not know how to cope with excessive saliva the result is that saliva may flow out. This should not be confused with salivation, which is a disease. The symptoms of salivation are increased amount of saliva flowing out from the mouth automatically. As the flowing of saliva goes on over a long period of time, the surrounding areas of the mouth, particularly the corner of the mouth, may flush and at times blister.

Massage Method

1. Commonly used manipulations

a. Let the child lie on its back. Rub the belly round and round clockwise with the palm of the hand for five minutes.

b. Let the child lie on its back. Push from Zhongwan to the navel on two sides with thumbs 20-50 times.

c. Cleanse Pijing 100 times and massage it for tonifying purpose 100 times. Knead Banmen 300 times.

d. Let the child lie on its belly. Press and knead Pishu and Weishu with the breadth of the middle finger for one minute each.

e. Press and knead Zusanli and Sanjianjiao for one minute each.

2. Additional manipulations

a. One kind of salivation is described as of the spleen and stomach insufficiency-cold type, indicated by the dribbling of thin saliva, pale face, cool limbs, thin stool, long urination, tasteless tongue and white and slippery tongue coating. The common manipulation to heal the disease is to cleanse Pijing 100 times. Massage Pijing 300 times for tonifying purpose. Pinch and knead Sihengwen 100 times. Knead Wailao 100 times. Push Sanguan 100 times. Knead Xiaotianxin 200 times.

b. Salivation of spleen and stomach qi-insufficiency type is characterised by the dribbling of thin saliva, sallow face, jaded appetite, fatigue, tasteless tongue, and thin and white tongue coating. To treat the case, cleanse Pijing 100 times. Massage it 300 times for tonifying purpose. Massage Feijing 300 times for the same purpose. Push Sanguan 300 times. Push Sihengwen 100 times. Massage Neibagua 100 times.

c. Spleen and stomach flaming heat type has symptoms, such as, dribbling of warm and sticky saliva, blistered mouth corners, thirst, halitosis, restlessness, constipation, scanty and dark urine, red tongue, and thin and yellow tongue coating. To deal with the case massage Pijing 100 times for tonifying purpose. Push Liufu 200 times. Cleanse Tianheshui 100 times. Cleanse Weijing 200 times. Knead Yongquan 100 times.

d. Salivation of the heart and spleen in gloom and depression type is marked by dribbling of warm and heavy sticky saliva, restlessness, red and stinking mouth, constipation, scanty and dark urine, red tongue, and thin and yellow tongue coating. The common manipulation to deal with the disease is to massage Pijing 100 times for tonifying purpose. Cleanse Xiaochang 300 times. Push Liufu 200 times. Cleanse Xinjing 200 times. Knead Xiaotianxin 100 times.

Suggested Regimen

a. Cultivate a good hygienic habit in the child. Remember always to keep the mouth cavity clean.

b. Primary diseases, such as facial paralysis and post encephalitis which develop into salivation should be duly treated.

Toothache

Toothache refers to pain in the tooth or teeth prompted by certain cause or causes. It is accompanied by pain in the gum as well. Children 7-8 years old may easily have tooth-ache, as milk teeth or deciduous teeth begin to fall away. Children may have bad habit in nibbling small bites between meals or before going to bed, or sleeping with candies or foodstuffs stuck in crevices between teeth. Clinical practices reveal that toothache aggravates when the child eats cold, hot, acid or sweet stuff, which stimulates into pain. This is ac-companied by feeling uncomfortable and fidgeting, mental fatigue, tiredness, no longer keen to speak, and loss of appe-tite.

Massage Method One

1. Commonly used manipulations
a. Let the child be placed in a seating position or lie down on bed. Knead Fengchi and Fengfu with the thumb or middle finger for one minute each.

b. Press and knead Hegu and Neiting on both sides for 1-3 minutes each.

c. Let the child be seated while the parent stands behind the child, pointing at and pressurising against Quepen on both sides with middle finger breadth. The parent should gradually relax the finger and press again. The process should be repeated 2-5 times.

d. Grip and lift up Jianjin 3-5 times slightly and softly.

2. Additional manipulations

a. Toothache and tooth swelling may be due to wind-fire. The pain is aggravated when the child takes hot or spicy food. Toothache alleviates when the affected tooth comes into contact with something cold. The gum is red and swollen. The child cannot chew food with its teeth. Other symptoms include swollen and hot cheeks, thirst, red tongue, and white and thin tongue coating. In addressing the problem the common manipulation is to press and knead Taiyang and Quchi acupoints for one minute each. Dip the bottom part of the palm in alcohol and rub the back of the child evenly for 1-3 minutes with the palm.

b. Toothache of the wind-cold type is indicated by slight pain in the gum at first. The pain aggravates and becomes acute. The child feels comfortable while eating something hot or warm. When the child is attacked by cold wind or drinks some cold beverage the pain aggravates. The child has an aversion to wind and cold. There is no thirst. The tongue is tasteless and red. The tongue coating is thin and white. The common manipulation is to grip and knead the muscular parts of the upper and lower limbs. Rub each limb with palm 3-5 times. Push the spealbone 100 times.

c. Toothache of the stomach-fire type is indicated by pain in the gum affecting the head and brain. The gum is swollen and red, affecting lips, tongue and cheeks. The face and eyes may become red. The child feels thirsty and wants to have cold drink all the time. The mouth is hot and stinks. The child is averse to warmth and prefers cold. Other symptoms include constipation, yellow urine, red tongue, and yellow tongue coating with little saliva. The common manipulation is to rub the belly counter clockwise for 3-5 minutes. Press and knead Zusanli and Sanyinjiao for one minute each. Press and knead Dazhui for one minute and rub the parts till they are warm.

d. Toothache due to deficiency fire is indicated by dull or slight pain, which increases in the afternoon. The gum is slightly red and swollen. In course of time the flesh in the gum becomes atrophic and the teeth floats as if in water. Lack of strength in chewing. The lips and cheeks are red. The throat is dry and in pain, followed by dysphoria and sleeplessness. There is an acrid pain in the hip and legs. The tongue is slightly red. The tongue coating is thin. The common manipulation to deal with the case is to rub Yongquan for 2-5 minutes. Rub Shengshu, Mingmen and the sacrococcygeal region till they are warm. Press and knead Taixi and Xingjian for one minute each.

Massage Method Two

1. Commonly used manipulations

a. Let the child lie on its back while the parent closes in on the forehead with two thumbs and rubs from centre to the sides repeatedly for one minute.

b. Press Taiyang with thumbs lightly at first and then heavily for one minute. Grip and lift up the muscle of the neck repeatedly for about one minute.

c. Slightly bend the five fingers of both hands. Spread out the fingers. Use strength of the finger tips to massage from forehead to the back of the head for 2-5 minutes.

d. Press and knead Xiaguan, Hegu and Neiting for one minute each.

e. Pinch and knead Zusanli, Sanyinjiao and Yongquan for

half a minute each.

2. Additional manipulations

a. For toothache in the upper teeth, press and knead Xiaguan, Yingxiang and Renzhong for one minute each.

b. For toothache in the lower teeth press and knead Hegu, Jiache and Yifeng for one minute each.

Suggested Regimen

a. Brush teeth after each meal.

b. Remove bad habit. Do not let the child sleep with the nipple in the mouth. Do not let the child eat candies before going to bed. Do not let the child eat nibbles between meals. Do not leave nipple in baby's mouth during sleep.

c. Protect the mouth cavity by avoiding stimulation to the teeth. Do not eat cold, hot, acid and sweet foodstuff.

Myopia

Myopia refers to inability to see distant things clearly, which is a common eye disease due to inappropriate use of the eye during youth or adolescence. The symptoms are blurred vision on seeing distant objects. The eyes see clearly objects that are near the person. If a child looks at something for a long time even at close range its eyes will swell or become bloated. There will be headache. The eyes will get tired. Myopia in extreme cases is characterised by protruding eyeballs.

Massage Method One

1. Commonly used manipulations

a. Let the child lie on its back. Push with thumbs from Yintang along the eyebrows to Taiyang for 1-3 minutes.

b. Let the child lie on its back. Rub lightly from inner eye corner via the lower eye sockets to Taiyang 10-20 times.

c. Press and knead Taiyang, Zanzhu, Jingming, Yuyao and Sibai for one minute each.

d. Press and knead Fengchi 10-20 times.

e. Let the child lie on its belly. Press and knead Xinshu, Ganshu and Shenshu for one minute each with the thumb.

2. Additional manipulations

a. For dry eyes and swollen and painful eye sockets the commonly used manipulations are to press and knead Shenshu and Ganshu for two minutes each. Press and knead Baihui 20 times. The commonly used manipulations of pressing and kneading Shenshu and Ganshu for two minutes should be further extended to more than three minutes. Massage Shenjing and Ganjing 300 times each for tonifying purpose.

b. For weak constitutions with deficiency of the spleen and stomach, press and knead Pishu and Weishu for one minute each. Rub Zhongwan 20 times. Press and knead Sanyinjiao for one minute.

Massage Method Two

a. Let the child lie on its back with eyes closed. Lightly press and knead the eyeball 10-15 times with the breadth of the thumb.

b. Press and knead Taiyang for two minutes.

c. Put the child in a seating posture. Press and knead

Fengchi for one minute with thumb and index finger. This is followed by pinching the muscle on both sides of the cervical vertebra from top to bottom 10-15 times.

d. Place the child in a seating posture. Rub from Yintang to both sides of the head with thumbs 5-10 times.

e. Grip Jianjin. Press and knead Xinshu and Ganshu for one minute each.

f. Put the child in a seated position. Bend fingers slightly and press and knead the scalp for one minute with finger tips. Comb and rub the hair of the child 10 times quickly.

Massage Method Three

a. Let the child lie on its back. Press and knead Jingming for 2-5 minutes with index fingers. Press and knead Zanzhui and Sibai 10-20 times each.

b. Let the child lie down with eyes closed. Lightly rub from inner eye corner to Taiyang along the upper part of the eyeballs with the breadth of thumbs 10-15 times.

c. Press and knead Taiyang for two minutes.

d. Put the child in a seating posture. Lightly press with thumbs and index fingers the auricle of the child till it is warm and red.

e. Press and knead Hegu, Zusanli, Fengchi and Yiming for one minute each.

Suggested Regimen

a. It should be remembered that massage yields good therapeutic results for pseudo near-sighted vision. In genuine myopia massage can only improve the vision.

b. Correct any improper use of the eye by the child. During reading or writing choose the right position to sit and the right position from which light comes from to protect the eyes.

c. Take exercise regularly—the sort of exercise that is designed to protect eyesight.

d. Do not touch eyes directly with fingers during massage.

Strabismus

Your optical axis or line of distance should be parallel as you look straight forward or turn to another direction. In looking squarely at something, if the optical axis does not centre on the same object (with one eye on the object but the other eye away from the object), then a person must be suffering from strabismus. The symptoms are that one eye remains slightly to the side of the nose or temple, which, however, does not impede the movement of eyeballs. In reading or looking at things in short distances the eyes look upward. Persons suffering from strabismus usually have poor eyesight in looking at both distant and near objects.

Massage Method One

1. Commonly used manipulations

a. Let the child who suffers from strabismus be seated or lie down. Knead from Yintang along one side of the eye socket for 1-3 minutes with the breadth of the thumb lightly and knead the other side of the eye socket for 1-3 minutes.

b. Put the tip of the index and middle fingers simultaneously on Jingming and turn round and round clockwise for one minute.

c. Press and knead Yuyao for one minute with the breadth of the thumb of both hands simultaneously.

d. Press and knead Taiyang for one minute with the breadth of middle fingers of both hands simultaneously.

e. Press and knead Sibai for one minute with the breadth of index fingers of both hands.

f. Grip and pinch Hegu 15-30 times.

g. Let the child lie down with eyes closed. Rub lightly from Jingming to Taiyang 50 times with the radialis of the thumb of both hands. Do not touch the eyeballs during manipulation.

h. Let the child lie on its belly. Press and knead Ganshu and Shengshu with fingers for one minute each.

2. Additional manipulations

a. If the child is in the grip of fever, convulsion and restlessness, press and knead Dazhui with fingers for one minute. Push and rub Yongquan 300 times. Rub the muscles on both sides of the spinal column with the bottom of the palm till diathermancy.

b. If the child with strabismus cannot see distant objects clearly and shows tiredness in looking at near objects with pain in eye socket and forehead, press and knead Fengchi for 1-3 minutes on the side of the eye in pain till there is a sense of fullness and heaviness conducted to the head. Massage Shenjing and Ganjing 300 times each for tonifying purpose.

Massage Method Two

a. Let the child sit or lie down. Press and knead Jingming, Chengxi, Sibai and Taiyang for one minute each with fingers. Rub the area surrounding the eye sockets with thumbs repeatedly for 1-3 minutes.

b. Let the child lie on its belly. Press and knead Ganshu, Danshu and Shenshu for 1-3 minutes each.

c. Pinch and knead Hegu and Guangming opposite the cross eye for 1-3 minutes each.

Suggested Regimen

a. Let the child rest and close its eyes. Reduce the degree of tiredness of the eye. Cut down the time in watching TV. Do not try to look at distant objects. Cut down the time in looking at near objects, such as playing with toys, building blocks or reading picture story books.

b. Acupuncture should be used alongside massage to raise the efficacy of therapy.

c. In case of hyperopia or long sight, the child should wear spectacles.

d. Alongside massage, normotopia may be undertaken to normalise the position of eyes in the child. In doing this use index fingers to lift up the front part of the eyes and push sideways. Let the child look around. Repeat the process many times. In course of time the eyes may become normal.

e. If the case is very serious and continues over a long period of time despite massage treatment, acupuncture or administration of medicine, the child should go through surgery at the hospital to correct the eyesight.

Stye

Stye, also known as hordeolum, is an acute inflammatory

disease in which the gland in the eyelid comes under attack by suppurative viruses. The symptoms are painful, red and swelling eyes. The red and swelling aggravate so much that the child is unable to open its eyes. The bacterial infection causes red small sore swelling to appear on the eyelids within a few days in most cases. Pus flows out from the eyes. The condition alleviates yet the disease usually lingers on over a rather long time.

Massage Method One

1. Commonly used manipulations

a. Place the child in a seating position or let it lie down on bed. Push up from Yintang to the hairline with the breadth of thumbs. The manipulation should be carried out alternately for 1-3 minutes.

b. Press Zanzhui for one minute with fingers. From Yintang push to Taiyang along the upper eyelids on two sides 10-15 times.

c. Press and knead Taiyang for one minute.

d. Press and knead lightly and softly the parts affected by the disease for 1-3 minutes with the breadth of the thumb.

e. Let the child be seated or lie on its belly. Press Fengchi on both sides with thumb and middle finger for one minute.

2. Additional manipulations

a. Stye of the wind-heat type due to attacks by external factors is characterised by slightly red, warm swelling eyelids, which prick, itche and become rather uncomfortable. The sore swelling assumes the shape of a wheat grain. Stye is accompanied by fever, aversion to wind, dry mouth, thirst, red tongue, and thin and yellow tongue coating. The common manipulation to heal the disease is to rub horizontal wise the medial side of the spealbone till it becomes warm. Press and knead Hegu and Quchi for one minute each. Cleanse Feijing 300 times. Cleanse Tianheshui 100 times.

b. Stye of the heat-poison full-hot type is indicated by swelling that becomes prominent with extreme pain. The swollen eyelids are accompanied by fever and thirst. The child is uncomfortable and fidgets. It suffers from constipation, scanty and dark urine. The tongue becomes red. The tongue coating is yellow. To deal with this case the common manipulation is to cleanse Tianheshui 300 times, cleanse Dachang 300 times and push Liufu 200 times. Press and knead Quchi, Hegu and Dazhui for one minute each. Rub Yongquan for 1-3 minutes. Push straight the muscles on both sides of the spinal column with the bottom part of the palm till they become warm.

c. Stye of the spleen and stomach heat full-hot type is characterised by red swollen eyelids, increased gum in the eyes, thirst and bitter taste in mouth, constipation, yellow and red urine, red tongue, and yellow tongue coating. The common manipulation to deal with this disease is: cleanse Weijing 200 times and Xiaochang 300 times. Cleanse Dachang 300 times. Push Liufu 300 times. Push Xiaqijiegu 300 times.

Massage Method Two

a. Press and knead Taiyang and Yintang for one minute each with fingers.

b. Pinch and press the bottom of the middle finger for 1-3 minutes with the thumb and middle finger.

c. Grip Fengchi and Jianjin 10-15 times each.

d. Let the child lie on its belly. Rub the lumbarsacral region with the bottom of the palm till diathermancy.

Massage Method Three

a. Press and knead Sanyinjiao for 1-3 minutes.

b. Pinch the middle toe in both feet 10-15 times each.

c. Let the child lie on its belly. Rub the back, hip and sacrum with the bottom of the palm till they are warm. Use empty fists to strike at the parts from top to bottom 10-20 times.

d. Press Quchi with the tip of thumbs first. Then pinch and knead the acupoint for 4-5 minutes with both thumbs alternately till there is an acid and swelling feeling.

Massage Method Four

a. Let the child clench fist and turn the fist upward. The parent pinches and kneads Houxi on both sides for 2-5 minutes with the thumb.

b. Let the child lie on its belly. Press and knead the medial side of the spealbone with the thumb 2-5 times.

c. Press and knead Taichong on either side for 1-3 minutes.

Suggested Regimen

a. Give hot compress treatment to the affected part of the eye in the initial period 3-4 times a day. Each treatment lasts 5 minutes. This will partly improve blood circulation in eyelids and absorption of oozings from inflammation. It will repair damaged tissues.

b. If pus comes out, do not try to press or squeeze it. Otherwise the pus may spread to other parts of the eye or to the brain, the consequences of which may be very serious.

c. Take hygienic measures to protect the eye. Do not use

hand or dirty towel to clean the eye.

    d. Take mild food. Do not eat greasy, spicy or hot stuff.

Spontaneous Sweating

Spontaneous sweating refers to sweating which occurs automatically. It is not caused by having taken diaphoretics, strenuous exercise, violent activities of one sort or another, hot weather, or wearing too many clothes. It occurs often among children with weak constitution. Clinical practice shows sweating occurs from time to time. Sweating aggravates due to bodily movement, accompanied by pale face, cool limbs, shortness of breath, lacking in strength and aversion to cold and wind.

Massage Method One

1. Commonly used manipulations

a. Massage Pijing and Feijing 300 times each for tonifying purpose.

b. Knead Shending for two minutes.

c. Knead Shenwen for one minute.

d. Let the child lie on its belly. Pinch the spinal column 5-10 times.

e. Pinch and knead Zusanli for one minute.

f. Press and knead Pishu and Feishu for one minute each.

2. Additional manipulations

a. Sweating due to disharmony in nourishment is indicated by automatic sweating, headache, aversion to wind, bad cold, running nose, aching all over the body, not thirsty, stomach not working properly, tasteless and red tongue, and thin and white tongue coating. Knead and lift up the muscle in four limbs. Rub each part 5-8 times with palm. Pinch and grip the muscle around Jianjin 5-10 times. Let the child lie on its belly. Push and rub with one palm the muscle on the sides of the spinal column till diathermancy.

b. Sweating of the qi-deficiency in spleen and lung type is characterised by automatic perspiration (particularly when the child is moving about), shortness of breath, cough, pale face, cool limbs, pale lips, catching cold easily, tasteless tongue, and thin and white tongue coating. The common manipulation to address the case is to push Sanguan 100 times. Knead Banmen 100 times. Rub Zhongwan for 2-5 minutes. Press and knead Danzhong and Sanyinjiao for one minute each.

c. Sweating known as of the stomach in flaming heat type is characterised by frequent perspiration in large quantities, thirst for cold beverage or water, high fever, red face, restlessness, dry stool, scanty and dark urine, red tongue, and yellow tongue coating. To deal with the case a common manipulation is to massage Pijing and Feijing 300 times each for tonifying purpose. Cleanse Tianheshui 200 times. Push Liufu 200 times. Cleanse Xiaochang 200 times. Push Xiaqijiegu 300 times.

Massage Method Two

a. Let the child lie on its back. Knead and rub Shenque clockwise for 2-5 minutes with the palm of the hand.

b. Use Xiaoyuji to knead and rub Guanyuan counter clockwise for two minutes.

c. Let the child lie on the belly. Push and rub the muscle

around Feishu and Dazhui for one minute each with the bottom of the palm.

d. Press and knead Zusanli and Fuliu for one minute each.

Suggested Regimen

There are four steps in this connection:

a. Nursing care should be stepped up. The child should change clothes more often than usual. Use a clean, soft piece of cloth to rub the body of the child to keep the skin dry.

b. Do not place the child in such a way that it is faced with wind blowing directly on its body to prevent the child from catching cold or from developing complications.

c. Let the child drink lots of water. Feed it with easily digestible food. Abstain from spicy, hot, greasy or sweet food.

d. In case the child sweats profusely, the doctor should be sent for. Otherwise the child may collapse.

Eczema

Eczema is a skin disease supersensitive to inflammation, common among babies. It is not a seasonal disorder, which may occur in any part of the body. Clinical practice reveals a skin condition in which areas of the skin may become red, rough and sore so that the baby wants to rub them—a recurrent skin eczema, such as papule, vesicle and pustule. The baby may have bouts of intense itching. It aggravates in the night and easily occurs again and again.

Massage Method One

1. Commonly used manipulations

a. Cleanse Feijing 300 times and cleanse Dachang 100 times.

b. Let the child lie down. Grip and lift up Baichong five times with thumb, index and middle fingers in a symmetrical or two-pronged manner.

c. Press and knead Quchi and Zusanli for one minute each.

d. Let the child lie on its belly. Knead with Xiaoyuji along the sides of the spinal column from Feishu downward to Pishu, Weishu, Sanjiashu, Shenshu and Baliao for five minutes. Press and knead simultaneously the above-mentioned acupoints.

2. Additional manipulations

a. Eczema of the damp and hot type is indicated by the presence of blebs all over the body, itching and burning. Other symptoms include restlessness, thirst, mental fatigue, constipation, scanty and dark urine, red tongue, and yellow and greasy tongue coating. The common manipulation to deal with this type of disease is to cleanse Xiaochang 300 times and push Liufu 100 times. Press and knead Yinlingquan and Sanyinjiao for one minute each.

b. Eczema due to over feeding with milk is characterised by scattered pimples, some of which itch, aversion to food, painful and swollen belly, acid stinking stool in semliquid form, constipation and thick and greasy tongue coating. The common manipulation to deal with the case is to press and knead Zhongwan for one minute. Knead Banmen 200 times. Massage Neibagua 200 times. Push Xiaoqijiegu 100 times.

Massage Method Two

a. Press and knead Quchi, Huantiao and Yanglingquan for one minute each with the breadth of the thumb.

b. Let the child lie on its belly. Grip and lift up the muscle around Geshu 10-20 times with thumb, index and middle fingers.

c. Press and knead Pishu, Weishu and Sanjiaoshu for one minute each.

d. Pinch and knead Zusanli and Sanyinjiao 20 times each with the thumb, and pinch Xuehai 50 times.

Suggested Regimen

a. Eczema is a protracted disease and may be recurrent. Apart from massage other therapies should be given, such as acupuncture, moxa-moxibustion and Chinese traditional and Western medicine (oral and externally administered).

b. Cultivate a normal life habit in the child. Avoid stimulation. Do not use hot water or too much soap to wash the child.

c. Do not eat greasy, hot and sweet food. Take only a bland diet.

d. Provide the child with good treatment during the acute stage to prevent the disease from becoming chronic.

Summer Heat

Summer heat is a special disease, which breaks out into

fever, among children below three years of age. It occurs mostly in hot summer days. The usual symptoms are, the child slowly gets sick. It has high fever which is unabated. The body temperature runs between 38-40 degrees Celsius for a period of 1-3 months. If the weather is hot, the body temperature rises. If the weather registers a lower temperature so does the body. The child is thirsty and drinks a lot of water. It passes water in large quantity. The urine is clear. The skin is dry. No or little perspiration. The face is pale. The body is lean and the constitution weakened due to high fever over a prolonged period of time.

Massage Method One

1. Commonly used manipulations

a. Cleanse Tianheshui 500 times and push Liufu 300 times.

b. Push Tianzhu 50-100 times from top to bottom with index and middle fingers.

c. Press and knead Dazhui for 1-3 minutes with fingers.

d. Let the child lie on its belly. Push with strength and rub the back and hip on the sides of the spinal column till diathermancy with Xiaoyuji of the hand.

e. Press and knead Zusanli for one minute.

2. Additional manipulations

a. Summer heat of the injured lung and stomach type is indicated by unabated fever (which rises in the afternoon), thirst, drinking a lot of water or beverage, dry skin, little or no perspiration, long, clear and light yellow urine, restlessness, red and dry lips, red tongue, and thin and white or thin and yellow tongue coating. The common manipulation to address the disease is to cleanse Feijing and Dachang 300 and 100 times respectively. Knead Xiaotianxin 100 times. Knead Zongjin 30 times. Knead Shenwen for one minute.

b. Summer heat of the intense upper part and weak lower part type is indicated by thirst, frequent urination with clear or yellow contents, no perspiration, depression and restlessness, pale face, jaded appetite, cool lower limbs, thin stool, tasteless tongue, and thin tongue coating. The common manipulation to heal this disease is to massage Pijing 300 times for tonifying purpose. Knead Banmen 300 times. Push and rub Yongquan 100 times. Rub Zhongwan for 2-5 minutes with the palm.

Massage Method Two

1. Commonly used manipulations
a. Cleanse Feijing 300 times. Push Liufu 300 times.

b. Knead Xiaotianxin 100 times. Cleanse Tianheshui 300 times.

c. Press and knead Pishu and Weishu with fingers for one minute each.

d. Push and rub Yongquan 100 times.

e. Pinch the spinal column 3-5 times.

2. Additional manipulations
a. Summer heat with accompanying exterior syndromes in the initial period may be cured by kneading Taiyang 30 times, pressing and kneading Quchi, Hegu and Dazhui for one minute each and lifting up and gripping Jianjing 3-5 times.

b. Summer heat of the injured qi type in the intermediate period can be treated by pressing and kneading Zusanli for one minute, kneading Neilaogong 100 times, pinching Zongjin five times, and pressing and kneading Dazhui for one minute.

c. Summer heat of deficiency of both qi and yin elments in the final phase of the disease may be cured by massaging

Pijing and Shenjing 300 times each for tonifying purpose, rubbing Zhongwan for five minutes with the palm, and pressing and kneading Zusanli for 1-3 minutes.

Suggested Regimen

a. The child should be confined to bed in a nice and cool place.

b. Vitamin-rich bland food should be provided, such as mung bean or rice congee, egg, green vegetables and fruits.

c. Keep the skin dry. Change clothing and bed sheet frequently. Diaper should be changed constantly in the case of younger children.

d. Do not let the child come into contact with other patients to prevent infection, since the child is weak and has low resistance to assault by infectious viruses.

e. Children suffering from high fever should be given cold treatment. Put a cold and wet towel on the head. Rub the child with alcohol. If necessary administer the child with medicine to bring down the fever or kill pain in accordance with the instruction of the doctor.

Obesity

Obesity refers to fat in the body in excess of the normal amount in a child as compared with children of the same age group and height. An obese child registers 20% more weight than normal. Clinical practice shows that the external appearance of an obese child is markedly very fat and tall. The development of bone structure in an obese child comes earlier than that of children in the same age group. The subcutaneous fat is very thick and distributed evenly. Fat is accumulated in an undue manner in cheeks, shoulders, chest, nipples and belly. The legs and upper arms are strong but the tip of limbs is rather thin. Blood pressure is normal or slightly higher than normal.

Massage Method One

1. Commonly used manipulations

a. Let the child lie on its back while the parent sits on the right side. Rub Zhongwan counter clockwise with Xiaoyuji of the right hand with some strength for five minutes.

b. Let the child lie on its back. Knead Tianshu clockwise on both sides with thumb and middle finger of the right hand for 1-3 minutes.

c. Place the child in the same position. Grip and lift up the muscles above and below the navel with thumbs, index and middle fingers. When you lift up the muscles, press and twist them. Put down the muscles gradually and slowly. Perform the operation 10-20 times.

d. Press and knead Qihai for one minute with the breadth of the middle finger.

e. Rub in the direction of the colon ascendens, descendens and transverse 10-20 times with the whole palm of both hands alternately.

f. Press and knead Zusanli and press and massage Fenglong for 1-3 minutes each. Pluck Hegu 10-15 times.

g. Press and knead Pishu and Weishu for one minute each.

2. Additional manipulations

a. An obese child who is short of breath and lacking in

strength should get additional treatment: Press and knead Danzhong for one minute. Pinch the spinal column 5-10 times. Rub the upper part of the chest horizontal wise till diathermancy. Massage Pijing 300 times and Feijing 100 times for tonifying purpose.

b. An obese child with constipation should get the following treatment: push Xiaqijiegu 300 times. Knead Guiwei for one minute. Press and knead the two sides of the body from armpit to the waist 30-50 times.

Massage Method Two

a. Let the child lie on its back. Press and knead Guanyuan clockwise and counter clockwise for five minutes each.

b. Let the child lie on its back. The parent, standing in front of the child, pushes from the heart to the pubic bone with one palm 10 times.

c. Let the child lie on its back. Press and knead the muscle of the four limbs for three minutes.

d. Press, knead and pluck Zusanli and Fenglong 20 times each.

e. Let the child lie on its belly. Pat two sides of the spinal column from top to bottom with empty fist 10-15 times.

f. Let the child lie on its belly. Rub the lumbosacral region with the entire palm till the region is permeated with radiant heat.

Suggested Regimen

a. The parent should be aware of the fact that an obese child does not enjoy good health. The calories injected to the child should be adequate to guarantee the normal development of the child. Extra calories are not warranted. This is to say that enough is enough.

b. Let the mother breast-feed the child for a minimum period of no less than three months. If a child cries, do not always feed it with milk. Crying does not necessarily mean that the child is hungry—it may cry for other reasons.

c. Feed the child that has a good appetite with bulky food containing less calories, such as vegetable and fruits. Where possible abstain from feeding the child with greasy, sweet or salty food.

d. Encourage the child to do physical exercise—walking, playing, slow-speed running and other light activities. Increase the amount and time of exercise gradually. Do not take exercise that increases appetite and requires intake of more food that will lead to more obesity.

Chilblain

Chilblain is an inflammation of part of the skin in winter or early spring caused by cold weather. It appears at the periphery of limbs or exposed parts of the body, such as hand, foot, tip of nose, side of ear, earlobe and cheeks. The symptoms in the early stage are swellings that are partially purple or red or hardened skin (the size of which is no more than that of a broad bean or finger nail), the borders of which are red, the centre is purple or blue. It is cold to the touch. If you press it the colour fades somewhat. It recovers somewhat slowly if pressure is removed from the chilblain. The swelling causes pain or a sense of fullness. It itches. If the chilblain comes into touch with something hot the sensation of fullness and itching will aggravate all the more. In serious cases blisters occur, which may rupture and become ulcer. The disease will drag on for a long time. It occurs far more easily in children whose circulation of blood in the tip of limbs is not good, whose limbs sweat easily or who suffer from chronic malnutrition. Usually it occurs in winter. As the weather gets warm the child may gradually recover.

Massage Method One

1. Commonly used manipulations

a. Kneading or rubbing may be undertaken on parts of the chilblain 5-10 times lightly and softly. The manipulator should avoid violent action in the course of massage.

b. Do not massage blisters or ulcers. Massage the parts that surround them. Massage blisters and ulcers when they have been healed and the blood is in full circulation.

c. Let the child lie on its back. Rub Guanyuan for 2-5 minutes with the palm counter clockwise. This is designed to warm the Yang element and dissipate the cold.

2. Additional manipulations

a. Press and knead Waiguan and Yifeng for one minute each on the child afflicted with chilblain in the ear. Rub the ear with thumb and index finger by applying considerable force for 2-5 minutes.

b. Press and knead Yingxiang for one minute on the child afflicted with chilblain on the tip of the nose. Grip Hegu for one minute. With thumb breadth lightly rub the nose till it becomes radiant with warmth.

c. Press and knead Hegu for two minutes on the child afflicted with chilblain on the face. This is followed by pressing and kneading Xiaguan and Jiache 20 times each. Rub the face with Dayuji till radiant heat.

d. Press and knead Quchi and Hegu for one minute each on the child afflicted with chilblain in the hand. Point at and pressurise Quepen for about one minute with the breadth of the thumb. Let go the hand slowly after manipulation. The child feels a warm sensation in the hand. Rub upper limbs with both hands horizontal wise for 1-3 minutes.

e. Press and knead Zusanli for one minute on the child afflicted with chilblain on the foot. Rub the sole of the afflicted foot with palm till a part of the sole becomes warm. Let the child lie on its side with legs apart, one leg in front and the afflicted one below. Pressurise the medial side of the leg with the bottom of the palm for one minute. Let go the hand slowly. The child now feels a warm sensation in the foot. Use the same method on the other leg.

Suggested Regimen

a. Do exercise and outdoor activities to strengthen the resistance of the child to cold.

b. See to it that the child does not catch cold. Put on more cloth on the child during changes in the weather. Let the child wear a mask on the mouth to prevent stimulation by cold wind. Do not let it go to the fireside at once when the child comes back to the room from outdoor. Warm the hands and feet gradually first and go to the fireside afterwards.

c. Administer Western or Chinese traditional medicine to the child that has serious chilblains or suffers from recurrent bouts of the disease. The medicine can be both orally administered or applied externally.

d. Feed the child in a reasonable way. Give it more nutrition to increase its power of immunisation.

e. Children suffering from chronic anaemia or are in a state of decline should receive prompt treatment.

Ankle Joint Sprain

This refers to spraining of joint or wrenching of joint with tearing or stretching of ligaments—a frequent illness encountered in the orthopaedics department in hospital. It occurs in persons of all ages. Children in secondary schools or in the age group for secondary schooling may sprain ankle most often, since they are most active during this period. The usual symptom is that the ankle bone is swollen and in pain. The patient cannot walk with the foot. The injured part has pressing pain. There is subcutaneous blood stasis in some parts of the foot. If the liagments in the ectocondyle are injured, the pain is obvious when the patient turns the foot towards the inside. In case the ligaments in the malleoulus medialis are injured, the pain is obvious when the patient turns the foot towards the outside. When ligaments are torn the patient can turn the foot inside or outside only in a lopsided manner and hematoma will break out.

Massage Method One

a. Let the child lie on its back. Press and knead Qiuxu, Taixi, Kunlun, Shenmai and Yanglingquan for half a minute each, lightly at first and heavily afterwards.

b. Stabilise the foot with one hand. Press and knead lightly and softly around the ankle joint with Dayuji of the other hand for 2-5 minutes.

c. Hold the toe with one hand and the heel with the other hand. Press the thumbs on the injured part and pull the hands downward with some force. Turn the ankle from inside to the outside and vice versa lightly for 1-3 minutes.

d. Hold the heel with one hand and the sole of the foot

with the other hand. In massaging the ankle joint, stretch it with strength. The manipulation should be carried out simultaneously. With strength stretch back the ankle joint. Turn round and round the joint for 1-3 minutes.

e. Apply strength with thumb and four fingers to grip and knead the ankle from top to bottom for 1-3 minutes. Rub the lower limb for one minute horizontal wise.

Massage Method Two

a. Let the child lie on its back. Rub lightly the injured part with Dayuji till diathermancy.

b. Use the breadth of the thumb to press and knead part of the injured ankle lightly and softly for 1-3 minutes.

c. Place the child in a seated position and hold its heel from the outer part. Press the thumb against the injured ligament while the other hand, holding the sole of the foot, shakes and swings it for one minute.

d. Hold the foot with both hands. Stretch and bend the sole. In pulling and pushing the foot, pressurise the injured ligaments with thumb by applying force for as long as the child can bear it. The manipulation is to last 5-8 minutes.

e. Press and knead the part below the knee joint and surrounding parts of joint of ankle bone with palms (using considerable force) for 2-5 minutes till they become warm with radiant heat.

Suggested Regimen

a. The patient with serious injured ankle bone joint should be X-rayed in the hospital to find out whether he/she has fracture or dislocation of the bone. If fracture has been established and diagnosed, the patient should be treated by a doctor.

b. During the acute period of ankle sprain, massage lightly, softly and slowly to avoid bleeding of the injured part. Do not give any hot compress treatment to the patient.

c. During convalescence massage more heavily. Hot compress treatment can be given to the patient in parts of the ankle. The injured ankle can be washed with traditional Chinese medicine to facilitate blood circulation and the flow of the main and collateral channels in which energy circulates. This often yields rather good results.

d. The injured part is kept warm or does not catch cold.

e. In the initial period the patient suffering from serious ankle sprain should not be allowed to make too many movements. In accordance with the condition of sickness he/she should rest in bed or on couch. After one or two weeks the patient can be told to move about and do some exercise to improve the function of the bone or ligament.

Rheumatoid Arthritis

Rheumatoid arthritis is a commonly seen chronic disease of the joint with accompanying symptoms that spread all over the body. It occurs more frequently among children of school age and particularly among females. During illness the joints in the entire body may be affected. The sickness strikes mainly at the small joints in the four limbs. In serious cases it may affect the spinal column and the sacroiliac joints. The symptoms are: low fever in the early stage of the disease, which manifests slowly. The muscles of the entire body become weak and limp. Loss of appetite and weight. The body becomes lean. At first the pain—— a sort of wandering pain, is felt in one or two small joints due to bodily movement. The joint becomes swollen and hardens. A part may become warm but not necessarily red. A typical case shows stiffness of joint in the morning during the initial period. Following the development of the disease the pain spreads from small joints to big ones, from a few to many. The pain may hit most joints. Atrophy of muscle occurs in late period. Deformity and tetanus occur when pathological changes take place.

Massage Method One

1. Commonly used manipulations

a. Let the child lie on its back. Put the hand on the belly and press and knead it clockwise for 2-5 minutes.

b. Grip and knead four limbs with thumb and four fingers (in particular, limbs and trunk). Press and knead the limbs and stretch the joints for 3-5 minutes.

c. Press, knead and pluck Zusanli with the tip of the thumb for 1-3 minutes.

d. Let the child lie on its belly. Rub the shoulder, back, hip, and sacrum with entire palm till diathermancy.

2. Additional manipulations

a. One type of ankle sprain is indicated by the child moving about in an unsettled manner. The injury is on joint in knee, ankle, elbow or wrist. The child has difficulty in stretching the joint. The pain is aggravated by wind. The tongue becomes tasteless and the tongue coating thin and white. The common manipulation to deal with this type of sprain is to press and knead Quchi and Hegu for 30 seconds each. Grip Fengchi for 10 seconds. Lightly pat the back of the child with empty fist for one minute.

b. Another type is characterised by acute pain, which is obvious in fixed places. The child has difficulty in stretching the ankle, which is cold in parts. When the child is in a warm place the pain alleviates. The pain aggravates when the child is in a cold place. The tongue is tasteless and tongue coating white. Rub the four limbs horizontal wise with palms, exerting considerable strength. Rub vertically spinal column and horizontally from armpit to hip. Keep on rubbing till diathermancy. Grip Jianjing 3-5 times.

c. The third type is characterised by heavy limbs, pain in muscle and joint, and limping movement. The child has difficulty in bending and stretching. The hip becomes cold. The feet suffer from edema. The stools are thin. The urine is abundant and clear. The tongue is tasteless and tongue coating white and greasy. Press and knead Jianjing and Hegu for 30 seconds each. Pat and strike with empty fist on either side of the spinal column from top to bottom till the skin is slightly red. Press and knead Pishu and Weishu for 30 seconds each.

d. The last is heat type, characterised by red, swollen and warm pain in the joint. When the patient is placed in a warm place the pain will be aggravated. The child has fever, thirst and dry throat. The face and eyes are red. The child is ill at ease and fidgets. The stool is dry. The urine is yellow. The tongue is red and tongue coating yellow or yellow and greasy. Press and knead Dazhui and Quchi for 30 seconds each. Pat and strike both sides of the spinal column with empty fists till they become somewhat red and warm. Grip Jianjing 3-5 times.

Massage Method Two

a. Let the child lie on its belly. Press and knead the sides of the spinal column from top to bottom 5-8 times till they ache and become swollen.

b. Press Dazhui, Feishu, Fengchi, Fengfu, Jianjing and Zusanli for 30 seconds-one minute respectively.

c. According to pathological changes and the sphere of activity, activate the joints: bend the joint of the shoulder forward, stretch backward, stretch outward, stretch inside and turn round; bend, stretch and shake the hip joint; and bend, stretch and extend the knee joint. Do not use violent force. Do it lightly, softly and slowly. Increase your strength gradually as you engage in these activities.

Massage Method Three

a. Let the child lie on its back. Use thumb and four fingers to grip and knead the upper limbs; at the same time coordinate the manipulation with the passive activities of joints from shoulder, elbow to wrist for 1-3 minutes. Press and knead Jianyu, Quchi, Zusanli and Hegu for 30 seocnds each.

b. Let the child sit down or lie on bed. Twist and knead wrist, breadth of each finger, and finger joint with the thumb and index finger. Shake them in a pertinent manner for 1-3 minutes.

c. Let the child lie on its back. Grip and knead the lower limbs from leg to ankle, which is co-ordinated with passive activities—bending, stretching, shaking and extending condyle and knee joint for 1-3 minutes. Press and knead Zusanli, Yanglingquan and Xiexi for half a minute each.

d. Press and knead the surrounding area of the knee joint with the bottom of the palm. Co-ordinate the manipulation with stretching, bending, turning inside and outside the joint. Twist and knead the podarthrum for 1-3 minutes.

Suggested Regimen

a. The child should be kept warm and provided with a diet that is rich in nutrition. Do not feed the child with cold food.

b. Rheumatoid arthritis is a chronic disease that lingers on over a long period of time. It is important to give it an early treatment. A suitable amount of exercise should be done by the patient. Do not over exhaust the patient.

c. Massage should be light, soft and gradual. Violent force is prohibited to avoid untoward consequences.

Keep-fit Massage for Children

Keep-fit massage for children has a long history. It does not cause pain and is welcomed by the children. Easy to comprehend, it can be mastered without much effort. It promotes fitness and development of children. The following are commonly used massages:

Ways to keep fit and strengthen the body

1. Manipulations

a. Massage Pijing 200-300 times for tonifying purpose.

b. Rub the abdomen for 2-5 minutes.

c. Pinch and knead Zusanli on either side 50-100 times each.

d. Pinch the spinal column 5-7 times.

e. Press and knead Pishu and Weishu 30-50 times each.

2. Points for attention

Manipulate once every day. Each course of treatment is 7 days. After one course take a rest for two days. Massage is given when the child has an empty stomach—before meal time.

Massage Method to Keep the Eyes Fit

1. Manipulations

a. With thumb push from Yintang to the front hairline, alternating the thumb 30-50 times. From the middle of the forehead rub sideways to Taiyang 30-50 times.

b. Press and knead Jingming, Zanzhu, Yuyao, Yangbai, Tongziliao, and Sibai 50 times each.

c. Let the child close its eyes. Press and knead the eyeball 20 times with the breadth of the thumb.

d. Press and knead Taiyang for one minute with the index finger.

e. Press and knead the eye socket 30-50 times.

2. Points for attention

This massage can be manipulated once a day. It can be used when there is eye strain resulting from looking at certain object over an unusually long time. For patients who are short-sighted the amount of massage can be increased.

Massage method to prevent common cold

1. Manipulations

a. Rub the palms quickly till they are hot. Put the hands on the forehead. Rub the face 50 times clockwise. Rub counter clockwise 50 times till the face is slightly red and has a warm sensation.

b. Push and rub both sides of the nose up and down

quickly with the index fingers. Do not exert too much strength during the manipulation. Stop the massage as soon as the nasal cavity has a warm sensation.

c. Knead and rub earlobes with thumb and index fingers for 1-3 minutes till the earlobes are red and warm.

d. Rub the shoulders and back with the entire palm till diathermancy.

e. Press and knead Hegu and Quchi 50 times each.

2. Points for attention

This massage can be used once a day. When flu is prevalent, the massage can be increased from one to three times. In addition to massage by parent, an older child may be taught to do self massage. Persistent massage will strengthen the body, prevent sickness and promote growth or physical development of the child.

(京)新登字 138 号
责任编辑：姜成安
　　　　　许　桁
封面设计：曾　磊

小 儿 按 摩

英文版

靳文龙　　林惠芳　　王淑翠

朝华出版社出版

中国北京车公庄西路 35 号　邮政编码 100044

中国国际图书贸易总公司发行

中国北京车公庄西路 35 号

北京邮政信箱 399 号　邮政编码 100044

1999 年第 1 版　　第 1 次印刷

ISBN 7-5054-0590-X/G·0168

03000

17-E-3267P

中华人民共和国印刷